The
Healthcare
C-Suite

Leadership
Development
at the Top

The
Healthcare
C-Suite

Leadership
Development
at the Top

Andrew N. Garman ▪ Carson F. Dye

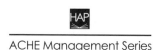

ACHE Management Series

13   12   11   10   09   5   4   3   2   1

Library of Congress Cataloging-in-Publication Data

Garman, Andrew N.
 The healthcare c-suite : leadership development at the top / Andrew N. Garman and Carson F. Dye.
  p. cm.
 ISBN 978-1-56793-313-0 (alk. paper)
 1. Health services administrators. 2. Leadership. I. Dye, Carson F. II. Title.
 RA971.G363 2009
 362.1068—dc22

                                                                    2009001020

The paper used in this publication meets the minimum requirements of American National Standard for Information Sciences—Permanence of Paper for Printed Library Materials, ANSI Z39.48-1984.∞™

Found an error or typo? We want to know! Please e-mail it to HAP1@ache.org, and put "Book Error" in the subject line.

For photocopying and copyright information, please contact Copyright Clearance Center at www.copyright.com or (978) 750-8400.

Project manager: Jane Calayag; Acquisitions editor: Eileen Lynch; Cover designer: Anne LoCascio

 Health Administration Press
 A division of the Foundation of the
   American College of Healthcare Executives
 1 North Franklin Street, Suite 1700
 Chicago, IL 60606-3529
 (312) 424-2800

To my wife, Deborah, who is everything to me,
and to our children, Emily and Tyler, my greatest source of
optimism for the future.

A humble "hats off" to the
clinicians and patients, whom our management profession was
created to serve.

—Andrew N. Garman

To my family—Joaquina, Carly, Emily, Liesl, Blakely, and Jeremy

A sincere salute to the many
fine, unsung leaders in healthcare—the ones who do not
get noticed.

—Carson F. Dye

Contents

Foreword

Having spent more than 40 years in healthcare, most of them in leadership roles in both clinical and administrative areas, I am extremely clear on this concept: Where we are successful, we have the right people in charge, and where we are failing, we have the wrong people in place. However, my four decades of experience have also taught me that most C-suite leaders are neither all good nor all bad and that, with commitment, outstanding leadership skills can be learned and refined over time.

The implications of these insights are addressed with wisdom and precision in Andy Garman and Carson Dye's newest book, *The Healthcare C-Suite: Leadership Development at the Top*. Garman and Dye truly recognize the complexity of healthcare management, which is exacerbated by the current global economic crisis.

Today, the healthcare industry is experiencing an almost perfect storm. Reimbursement is declining, regulations are increasing, morale among service providers is low, and supply costs are rising. In addition, more and more experienced CEOs are leaving their roles, often before they reach retirement age and sometimes because of the stress. The demand for outstanding healthcare leadership has never been greater. Consequently, the need for leadership development, talent management, and succession planning has never been more critical.

Recognizing that the quality of leadership is a key success factor for any healthcare organization, Garman and Dye developed key and meaningful assumptions essential in driving the leadership development process. They argue that leadership development, done well, is a long-term investment that yields a high rate of return (which is demonstrated and measured by performance improvement) and ultimately leads to outcomes that are at least as valuable as the time investment it requires. In short, just like clinical operations, leadership development needs to be not only efficient but also evidence-based.

As it does with many other management practices, the private sector has leadership development down to a science. The healthcare management community also must take notice, and it seems to be starting to do so. For example, CAHME (Commission on Accreditation of Healthcare Management Education), the accrediting body of healthcare administration programs, now requires all accredited programs to take a competency-based approach. In my capacity as chair of CAHME's board and its standards committee, I have supported these changes as necessary and helpful to the evolution of the profession. Healthcare delivery will continue to grow in complexity, as new technologies are devised, old illnesses are cured, and new diseases are discovered. Thus, both the development and practice of leadership competencies are imperative now. Excellence in healthcare leadership will mean a serious commitment to lifelong learning, using the strategies and tools articulated in this book.

Leadership training and development must be supported at the top—by the CEO, the COO, and other senior executives. These leaders must recognize and reaffirm every day that outstanding leadership talent is critical to the success, quality, and sustainability of healthcare delivery. That is what our patients, who entrust their lives to us, deserve.

Thomas C. Royer, MD
Chief Executive Officer, CHRISTUS Health

Preface

Consider the following scenarios common in the C-suites of today's hospitals and healthcare organizations.

1. A chief executive officer (CEO) directly supervises a 55-year-old vice president (VP). Having worked at the organization for many years, the VP has a track record of success. However, his skills are clearly deficient in some areas—in particular, he continuously leaves key people out of decision making, and he has a tough time admitting when his decisions are wrong. The CEO wonders if this person can be developed at this late stage of his career.

2. A CEO manages an exceptionally bright 35-year-old chief financial officer (CFO), who is a strategic thinker, outstanding at financial analysis, and brilliant at developing financial forecasts. This CFO, however, tends to push the financial agenda too strongly and does not seem aware of how she comes across to people who do not share her priorities. The CEO knows she can be developed but is unsure of the best approach to take: Should she be sent to a professional development class, paired up with an executive coach, or assigned a project that will push her to improve her interpersonal style?

3. For the past eight years, a chief operating officer (COO) has worked under the CEO. With her retirement only two years away, the CEO is beginning to realize that she has not fully developed the COO, who expects to be named as her replacement. Several board members have candidly expressed to the CEO their concern that the COO is not ready to fill the chief executive role. What should the CEO do?

4. Because of frequent CEO turnover at his organization, a VP has reported to three different CEOs in the last five years. The VP has less-than-satisfactory leadership skills, but none of his former supervisors confronted him about his underperformance. The current CEO is preparing to have that difficult discussion. She is considering several approaches—should she focus only on the VP's performance, or should she also look into the gaps in the system that allowed this development problem to continue unchecked for so long?

C-suite and senior leadership is qualitatively different from management at other levels. As such, professional development at this executive level requires a different approach. Unfortunately, as depicted in these scenarios, leadership development at this level tends to be driven by immediate rather than strategic needs. Often, executive leaders recognize the potential talent among their staff only when they are seeking to fill a position, and by that time, it is too late for much meaningful development. Also, many executives spend little time guiding direct reports to understand their own strengths and weaknesses, leaving the onus of professional development in the hands of the individual leader. These missteps result in haphazard development, ongoing blind spots, and unrealized internal leadership potential.

Senior executives themselves seldom pursue continuing education related to leadership competency development. Often, the scant leadership development they get comes from attending annual meetings of their professional societies. When they do go to in-house leadership development programs, in which their middle managers are also present, these executives are guarded, hesitant to fully participate in exercises and competency assessments. Because many senior-level performance evaluations focus only on *what* was achieved (e.g., higher revenue, improved clinical outcomes, better patient/physician/employee satisfaction) and not on *how* it was accomplished (e.g., collaboration/teamwork, mutual respect, good recruitment and retention strategies), bad habits and a misguided mind-set about self-development can continue unchallenged for years.

The levels of complexity and uncertainty in healthcare today are unprecedented and overwhelming. The challenges we will face in the coming years will require true systems change. They will demand that leaders from different professions and departments work together to support this evolution while minimizing collateral damage. Clearly, the old training model of sending people off on their own to a conference or seminar will not take organizations where they need to go.

ABOUT THIS BOOK

The Content

In *Exceptional Leadership: 16 Critical Competencies for Healthcare Executives* (HAP 2006), we describe the key knowledge, skills, and abilities most closely associated with extraordinary leadership at the executive level. The book serves as a personal guide for development, offering strategies for assessing and enhancing one's competencies and for finding mentors.

While *Exceptional Leadership* focuses on how you can improve your own performance, this new publication—*The Healthcare C-Suite: Leadership Development at the Top*—guides you in helping other leaders (specifically, the senior management team) harness, strengthen, and optimize their talents and capabilities. Of course, the concepts presented here can also apply to your own development needs.

If you are serious about your team's professional development, this book is for you. Not only does it lay out the most effective approaches to leadership improvement, it also offers strategies for overcoming common, but not so straightforward, barriers to learning. In addition to tapping our broad experience working with healthcare leaders, we digested the best current research and thinking on each subject we cover. We present this material clearly and succinctly, as we understand that time is often your tightest resource and thus must be invested with great care.

Although this book is a useful guide, it is not a magic pill that will cure all your leadership aches and pains. It is more a treatment regimen that needs to be followed with discipline and dedication. Building leadership talent does not happen overnight. Doing so is a gradual process, and that process is laid out in this book.

The Audience

While much of this book has relevance to managers at all levels, it was written specifically with senior executives in mind. C-suite leaders set the continuing education and development tone for the rest of the organization. As such, they should be models for life-long learning, not continually struggling to include professional development in their agenda.

This book is particularly applicable to the following groups:

- C-suite executives (CEOs, COOs) who aim (1) to develop their entire senior management team or a problematic leader and (2) to bring sophistication to their middle-management development process
- Vice presidents who seek to bring out the best in their leadership teams

- Coaches and consultants who help healthcare leaders achieve higher levels of performance
- Senior leaders who want to advance their skills in developing in-house talent
- Faculty and instructors in management and administrative programs who want to give their students an understanding of best practices in leadership development

The Structure

The book is organized in three parts.

Part I provides the foundation. Chapter 1 presents a useful approach to identifying leadership traits and talent. Chapter 2 summarizes the sources of motivation for leaders generally and for superb leaders particularly. Chapter 3 examines the position, career, and life stages that influence a leader's development. Chapter 4 describes how the leadership learning process takes place through the work leaders do. Here, we describe the three factors in workplace learning: tasks and assignments, feedback, and learning orientation.

Part II shows how the concepts in Part I are applied. Chapter 5 introduces a structured approach and tool, called the Developmental Interview, for formulating a focused, on-the-job development plan. Chapter 6 makes a case that development should be viewed as an investment that requires a change in mind-set, support, constant monitoring, and incorporation into daily organizational work. Chapter 7 focuses on derailment, offering methods for identifying early warning signs and intervening swiftly and appropriately. Chapter 8 addresses leadership transitions, providing strategies for facilitating effective passages, not just for your leaders but also for yourself. Chapter 9 expands the development dialogue from the individual to the broader organization.

Part III considers the common challenges in leadership development. Chapter 10 reviews the difficulties faced by diverse (or minority) leaders. Chapter 11 examines the dynamics of age and tenure, including the generation gaps between leaders and their direct reports (or vice versa). Chapter 12 discusses "delicate transitions"—movements from one position to another that require careful navigation—including from clinician to manager and from manager to executive. Chapter 13 presents the compelling case that personal growth and renewal are essential to lifelong leadership excellence.

Three appendixes conclude the book. Appendix A is an example of the Developmental Interview Guide discussed in Chapter 5. Appendix B is a grid for identifying development assignments that match the competencies to be developed. Appendix C is an annotated listing of healthcare organizations and associations that provide continuing education programs.

OUR LEADERSHIP DEVELOPMENT PHILOSOPHY

The practice of developing leaders is based on the following three assumptions:

1. Leadership development is a long-term investment that requires short-term sacrifices.
2. Leadership development is a relatively safe investment that yields a return in the form of improved performance across the leadership team.
3. Returns on these leadership investments tend to compound over time.

In our experience, leaders who commit to development almost always find these assumptions to be true. Indeed, if these premises were false, little or no leadership development would take place anywhere within the private sector, let alone in healthcare.

Also, experience has taught us that many senior executives in healthcare relegate the responsibility of leadership development to the chief human resources officer or the organizational development staff. This is *not* the approach taken by organizations in the private sector. In those settings, leadership development is a line function, often seen as one of the most critical activities undertaken by senior management.

Your reading of this book indicates to us that you are serious about developing your leaders. We applaud you for that and for recognizing development as a core part of excellent leadership.

Andrew N. Garman   *Carson F. Dye*

Acknowledgments

Andrew N. Garman's Acknowledgments

Most of what I know about leadership does not come from my own experience, but rather from the wisdom that healthcare leaders have shared with me. Sometimes this insight is offered to me by participants in interviews and graduate courses; other times, it arises from my occasional role as a sounding board, a position I am privileged to be asked to take from time to time. In both counts, I am extremely fortunate that in the last ten years I have had the opportunity to work at Rush University Medical Center, an organization that is a magnet for accomplished leaders who hold in high regard the value of reflecting on experience and who generously share their experiences.

To this end, I acknowledge the role that the leaders at Rush in general and the practitioner-faculty of the health systems management department in particular have played in deepening my understanding of leadership in healthcare. All of these people have shaped my knowledge in ways too many to list.

I am grateful to several leaders who had a particularly direct impact on this book. First on the list is Peter Butler, who chairs Rush's health systems management department when he is not busy running a world-class academic medical center. Not far behind are Bob Clapp, Brian Smith, Sheri Marker, and Jane Grady, all of whom I have reached out to on numerous occasions for their perspectives on senior leadership.

A special thanks also to the role-model leaders who have contributed to the governance, interprofessionalism, and leadership courses that I co-teach with Armen Galluci and Dr. Robert S. Higgins. They are Dr. Ross Abrams, Paola Cieslak, Courtney Kammer, Dr. Larry Goodman, Christina Jack, Diane McKeever, Avery Miller, Dr. Guy Petruzzelli, Brian Smith, Marie Sinioris, and Alison Walsh. When these talented individuals grace our class, I find myself taking as many notes as our students. My gratitude also goes to Lauren Brinkmeyer, director of the Rush administrative fellowship program and a highly involved faculty member. I can always count on her to make anything we collaborate on even better.

The faculty and staff that compose the core of the health systems management department at Rush also deserve acknowledgment: Dan Gentry, Diane Howard, Tricia Johnson, Mary Odwazny, Pat Pavia, Shital Shah, Frank Phillips, and Leslie Compere. I find inspiration in their own pursuit of excellence.

The health administration education community is vibrant and highly collegial, and I am fortunate to hear from faculty and students who have run into my work as part of their education and research. Their feedback has inspired me to keep working on these subjects, and it has also helped me better understand what is most helpful from a learning perspective. I want to particularly thank Dr. Louis Rubino, professor and director of the program at California State University, Northridge. Every year, he seems to rise on the shortlist of people I contact when I need some perspective. I also want to thank Dick Kilburg, David Leach, John Lloyd, Ann McAlearney, Dr. Tom Royer, and Larry Tyler—all of whom have strongly influenced my thinking about leadership education and development. Thanks as well to Joyce Anne Wainio, Judith Calhoun, and our colleagues in the NCHL demonstration project.

Few people can write without disrupting their home front. I want to deeply thank Deborah, my wife, and our children—Emily and Tyler—for their support, endurance, and tolerance while I visited the library on the sunniest days of the summer. Thanks also to my parents and grandparents for instilling a strong familial culture of rigorous critical thought and a keen respect for scientific inquiry.

Tremendous thanks to the entire staff of Health Administration Press, and a particular thanks to Jane Calayag, who has an uncanny knack for finding ten words that fit just fine in place of the hundred or so we provide her, and to Audrey Kaufman, who gave the initial green light for this project.

Last, and certainly not least, I deeply appreciate Carson's support and encouragement to pursue this book with him. I am grateful for the opportunity to continue our working relationship and benefit again from the wisdom of his considerable experience. While he will undoubtedly suggest I carried more "water," without his encouragement I would not have picked up the bucket in the first place. Thanks.

Carson F. Dye's Acknowledgments

This is my second book with Andy Garman, and I must say that working with him continues to be gratifying. In this new endeavor, Andy "carried most of the water," so to speak. His vast contribution to the content definitely has to be acknowledged. Our partnership is based on our mutual interest in healthcare leadership and how it is assessed and developed. Andy brings balance to our work: He not only understands the academic and research aspect of leadership, but he also has a grasp of how these principles apply in day-to-day operations. That's a rare thing to find. As he had done in our earlier collaboration, he set good timetables and kept me on task. Andy, it was great to work with you again; thanks much!

With humility, I must acknowledge the laboratory in which I work. Executive search gives me incredible opportunities to observe, study, and assess leadership. Almost every day, I meet excellent leaders who have accomplished outstanding results. Walking into some of the finest healthcare organizations in the world and gaining an in-depth perspective from their leaders have been an honored privilege. My clients, candidates, and placements have taught me much, and together we continue to work hard to make healthcare a better place.

I am grateful to many individuals whose leadership styles and approaches have had a powerful impact on me: Sister Mary George, Mark Hannahan, Mike Gilligan, Mike Covert, Gretchen Patton, Mike Doody, and John Thornburgh. Thanks also to these exemplary leaders: Steve Mickus, Scott Malaney, Bill Linesch, Dr. Scott Ransom, Dr. Greg Taylor, and Tim Sughrue. Many more leaders deserve acknowledgment, but our limited space does not permit me to enumerate all of their names.

I am very appreciative of the following individuals who helped so much with our diversity chapter—Howard Jessamy, Oliver Tomlin, Judson Allen, Walter McLarty, Barbara Palmer, Steve Yamada, and Michelle Taylor-Smith.

The Health Administration Press staff are top-notch. I am indebted to Audrey Kaufman, who got us started on this project. While she deserves a restful retirement, she is missed. I also appreciate Jane Calayag, who did a great job editing our final version. Health Administration Press provides a great service to our profession and the industry. I am so thankful that we have such a fine publisher.

As I have done in prior books (and in private), I offer a heartfelt note to my family. Joaquina, my wife, has been a tremendous foundation and supportive backer for more than 35 years now. She is enormously responsible for my successes. My daughters—Carly, Emily, Liesl, and Blakely—continue to be so encouraging. They missed many chances to be with me as I was out traveling and learning about leadership in healthcare. My family makes me who I am.

PART I

CHAPTER 1

Defining Talent

Robert is the new CEO of a large, multihospital health system, where he has worked for the last 18 years. Starting at the system's flagship hospital as a financial analyst, he quickly moved up within the finance department and later filled a line operations position. After several more career advances, Robert became the COO and then a CEO of one hospital in the system, his final roles before being tapped for the system-CEO duties.

Robert is hosting his first retreat for the entire senior leadership team. The theme of the retreat is leadership development and talent management. Following are Robert's opening remarks.

"Thanks for your support over the past few weeks as I began my new role. In the coming months, we will continue our work on the new strategic vision for the system, locking down the specifics of how we will invest in our future. For today, though, we are not here to discuss operations, trends, or investments. Instead, we will talk about how to ensure that all of us, including the leaders who report to us, will prove capable of handling the tasks and responsibilities associated with achieving that new strategic vision.

"I call this process 'talent management.' Others may refer to it by different names, but the basic idea is the same. We need to precisely define our meaning of leadership talent, not just now but also in the next five years, so that we can appropriately evaluate performance and communicate and manage this shared understanding. Our goal today is to establish a leadership definition and a model for talent management.

"Of course, leadership is different at various levels. We will accommodate these differences in our model. For today, though, our facilitator is here to focus our discussion on senior management.

Although we will not have the model fully polished by the end of the day, we should come away knowing that we are moving in the right direction, with a clear plan for finishing the work in the coming weeks. From there, we will move to embed our competencies into our leadership promotion and succession processes."

IN THIS VIGNETTE, the new CEO is focused not just on *what* but also on *how* the future strategic direction will be followed. Most important, he raises the visibility and emphasis on leadership development. By approaching talent management at the highest level, the CEO is allowing this effort to easily permeate the rest of the system.

Before we can develop leadership talent, we must first clearly define talent or the aspects of leadership that are associated with high performance. In this chapter, we offer several ways to identify these characteristics, including the Nine-Box Technique and leadership competencies.

THE NINE-BOX TECHNIQUE

Originally developed and used by General Electric, the nine-box approach is now widely used in many industries, including healthcare. This technique is a simple first step to defining talent in that it allows leaders to categorize performance levels for a group of managers. The approach involves the following:

1. *Identify a group of employees.* You may select your direct reports or all employees within the department or division.
2. *Place each employee name into the nine-box matrix* (shown in Figure 1.1). The matrix is divided into three performance levels—excellent, good, and fair—related to an employee's "current performance" and "future potential."

Figure 1.1 The Nine-Box Matrix

Current Performance
(How does this employee currently achieve results and perform his/her responsibilities?)

		(−) Fair (+)	(−) Good (+)	(−) Excellent (+)
Future Potential *(How does this employee demonstrate his/her capabilities for a promotion?)*	Excellent	III.	II.	I.
	Good	IV.	III.	II.
	Fair	V.	III.	III.

Group I: Exceptional Leaders. These employees are the potential future leaders of the organization.

Group II: Distinguished Performers. These employees are potential future leaders who have demonstrated one or several competency limitations.

Group III: Solid Performers. These employees are essential partners to Distinguished Performers and Exceptional Leaders.

Group IV: Questionable Performers. These employees perform at acceptable levels but never go above performance standards.

Group V: Problem Performers. These employees perform and behave poorly. They need constant supervision, instruction, and correction, drawing away needed talent from critical areas.

Source: Adapted with permission from APQC. 2001. "The Matrix: A Tool for Succession Management." [Online information; retrieved 6/1/08.] www.apqc .org/portal/apqc/ksn/TheMatrix.pdf?paf_gear_id=contentgearhome&paf_dm= full&pageselect=contentitem&docid=107003. For more information, contact www.apqc.org.

As with other performance appraisals, leaders approach the Nine-Box Technique differently—that is, they use varying definitions for "excellent," "good," and "fair." Thus, you should clarify the expectations for each performance level before embarking on this exercise.

Classifying Current Performance Levels

In considering an employee's performance in a current position, first determine what the job is designed to accomplish, according to the job description. In our definition, a good performer is someone who is delivering on all parts of the job effectively. An employee who is underperforming in one or more areas may be considered a fair performer at best. If an employee is "raising the bar"—not only doing his defined job well but also accomplishing goals above and beyond his role—that employee may be considered an excellent performer.

In using the Nine-Box Technique to evaluate current performance, you may find that many employees fit into the gray areas of performance between the three distinct categories (excellent, good, or fair). As such, leaders may find it difficult to assign employees "cleanly" into one or another performance level. This can be particularly hard when the technique is used for a large number of employees, where two individuals may be considered "good" performers despite the fact that one of them can use a little improvement but does not quite fall into "fair." What is helpful in this case is to add a plus/minus designation to each performance category. For example, Employee A's overall performance is solid, but he occasionally misses critical deadlines or fails to include key players in his decision-making process. With a plus/minus designation, Employee A can be rated as "good (–)," indicating that his performance is not on par with the "good (+)" employees.

Determining Future Potential

Assessing future potential can be even trickier than categorizing current performance. Two considerations can make this process more straightforward:

1. *Where does the employee fit within the organizational structure?* You can determine the individual's future potential in terms of career path or advancement. What is the likelihood that this employee will be promoted to a higher position?
2. *What does the employee need to be successful at his or her next role?* Consider the person's skills *and* motivation. What are the job expectations (skills, knowledge, and abilities) for the next role? Is this person focused on or working toward career advancement and success?

An employee with a high level of motivation and demonstrated relevant skills has "excellent future potential." Similarly, someone who is not as ambitious but delivers strong current performance (or vice versa) can be considered to have "good future potential." An individual who has either low motivation or low current performance generally falls under the "low future potential" category.

Evaluating Your Own Judgment

The next step is to use the results of the Nine-Box Technique to help you define talent. Here are useful questions to consider:

How confident am I in my judgments? Some employees' performance and potential are easier to pinpoint than others'. Judging these elements tends to become less complicated as the leader gains greater familiarity with the exercise and more opportunities to observe staff performance. If you are not confident about your categorization, think about specific moments or tasks that involved the employees you have identified for this exercise. Use these "critical incidents" to anchor and refine your perspective and judgment.

How do my views compare with others? The Nine-Box Technique can give you a sense of how strict or lenient you are in assessing performance. In our experience with organizations that have used this model, usually about 10 percent to 20 percent of employees fall into the Exceptional Leader and Distinguished Performer categories. Similarly, at least 10 percent to 20 percent of employees typically belong in the Questionable Performer and Problem Performer groups. So if you rated half of your staff as "exceptional" or "distinguished," and almost no one was assessed as "questionable" or "problem," you need to set a higher bar for solid or high performance. Conversely, if no one was placed into the Exceptional or Distinguished categories, your standards are probably too high.

Are the expectations for excellent, good, or fair performance clear and communicable? Even if the categories are understandable to you, they may not be clear enough to everyone else. Your direct reports will only benefit from this exercise and your judgment if they know what specific behaviors and actions are associated with success. Articulating these details is a struggle for most leaders; they can recognize excellent work when they see it, but they find describing what they see to be much harder.

Fortunately, numerous competency models have emerged that can help you communicate the what, how, and why of outstanding performance. In fact, many organizations have established their own models for this purpose.

LEADERSHIP COMPETENCIES

Competencies are developed to create a common language for understanding performance standards. The term "competency," however, means different things to different people. For this book, we use the following definitions (Dye and Garman 2008):

- *Competencies* are employee characteristics that lead to behaviors that are associated with high leadership performance.
- *Competency model* is an integrated framework of competencies.
- *Core competencies* refer to a set of competencies that apply to all positions (i.e., not specific to a given job or job family) and are associated with high organizational performance.
- *Competency modeling* is a systematic process for identifying and articulating competencies at one or more levels (individual, team, job family, or organization).

"Competence," although similar sounding, is not the same as "competencies." Competence is the *minimum* ability to perform a task or role (often clinical roles). In contrast, competencies are used to describe *higher* levels of performance. That is, a person may need to improve in one or more competency areas, but he or she is nonetheless competent in the role.

As we explore in more detail in Chapter 2, the motivation of excellent leaders tends to be different from that of their peers. Competency models are particularly helpful in engaging these senior managers because these models address the motivations of exceptional leaders.

The Exceptional Leadership Competency Model

Our book *Exceptional Leadership* presents 16 competencies that distinguish top performers from strong performers (Dye and Garman 2006). Following is a summary of these 16 competencies.

Cornerstone One: Well-Cultivated Self-Awareness
1. *Living by personal conviction* means you know and are in touch with your values and beliefs, are not afraid to take a lonely

or unpopular stance if necessary, are comfortable in tough situations, can be relied on in tense circumstances, are clear about where you stand, and will face difficult challenges with poise and self-assurance.

2. *Possessing emotional intelligence* means you recognize personal strengths and weaknesses; see the linkages between feelings and behaviors; manage impulsive feelings and distressing emotions; are attentive to emotional cues; show sensitivity and respect for others; challenge bias and intolerance; collaborate and share; are an open communicator; and can handle conflict, difficult people, and tense situations effectively. Emotional intelligence is often labeled EQ (emotional intelligence quotient).

Cornerstone Two: Compelling Vision

3. *Being visionary* means that you see the future clearly, anticipate large-scale and local changes that will affect the organization and its environment, are able to project the organization into the future and envision multiple potential scenarios/outcomes, have a broad way of looking at trends, and are able to design competitive strategies and plans based on future possibilities.

4. *Communicating vision* means that you distill complex strategies into a compelling call to act, inspiring and helping others see a core reason for the organization to make a change; discuss issues beyond day-to-day tactical matters; show confidence and optimism about the future of the organization; and engage others to join in.

5. *Earning loyalty and trust* means you are direct and truthful; are willing to admit mistakes; are sincerely interested in the concerns of others; show empathy and a generally helpful orientation toward others; follow promises with actions; maintain confidences and disclose information ethically and appropriately; and conduct work in open, transparent ways.

Cornerstone Three: A Real Way with People

6. *Listening like you mean it* means you maintain a calm, easy-to-approach demeanor; are patient, open minded, and willing to hear people out; understand others and pick up on their meaning; are warm, gracious, and inviting; build strong rapport; see the real meaning behind words others express; and maintain formal and informal channels of communication.

7. *Giving feedback* means you set clear expectations, bring important issues to the table in a way that others "hear" them, show an openness to facing difficult topics and sources of conflict, deal with problems and difficult people directly and frankly, provide timely criticism when needed, and offer clear and unambiguous feedback.

8. *Mentoring others* means you invest the time to understand the career aspirations of your direct reports; work with direct reports to create engaging mentoring plans; support staff members in developing their skills; encourage career development in a non-possessive way, allowing staff to move up or out as necessary; present stretch assignments and other demanding responsibilities; and pursue professional development to be a role model to others.

9. *Developing teams* means you select executives who have a team orientation, actively support group work, encourage open discourse and healthy debate on important issues, create compelling reasons and incentives for teamwork, set limits on the political activity that takes place outside the team framework, celebrate successes with the team, and commiserate as a group over disappointments.

10. *Energizing staff* means you set a personal example of good work ethic and motivation; talk and act enthusiastically and optimistically about the future; enjoy rising to new challenges; take on your work with energy, passion, and drive to finish successfully; help others recognize the importance of their

work; are enjoyable to work for; and have a goal-oriented, ambitious, and determined working style.

Cornerstone Four: Masterful Execution

11. *Generating informal power* means you understand the roles of power and influence; develop compelling arguments or points of view based on your knowledge of others' priorities; establish and maintain useful networks up, down, and sideways in the organization; develop a reputation as a go-to person; and directly and indirectly influence the thoughts and opinions of others.

12. *Building consensus* means you frame issues clearly and from multiple perspectives, separate issues from personalities, skillfully use group decision methods (e.g., nominal group technique), draw quieter group members into discussions, find shared values and common adversaries, and facilitate discussions rather than guide them.

13. *Making decisions effectively* means you make decisions based on an optimal mix of ethics, values, goals, facts, alternatives, and judgments; use decision tools (e.g., force-field analysis, cost-benefit analysis, decision trees, paired comparisons analysis) effectively and at appropriate times; and have good timing related to decision making.

14. *Driving results* means you mobilize people toward greater commitment to a vision, challenge people to set higher standards and goals, keep people focused on achieving goals, give direct and complete feedback that keeps teams and individuals on track, quickly take corrective action as necessary to keep everyone moving forward, show a bias toward action, and proactively work through performance barriers.

15. *Stimulating creativity* means you see broadly outside of the typical, are constantly open to new ideas, are effective with creativity group processes (e.g., brainstorming, nominal group technique, scenario building), are alert to future trends and can craft responses to them, are knowledgeable in business

and societal trends, know how strategies play out in the field, are well read, and make connections between industries and unrelated trends.

16. *Cultivating adaptability* means you quickly see the essence of issues and problems, bring clarity to ambiguous situations, approach work using various leadership styles and techniques, track changing priorities and readily interpret their implications, balance consistency of focus with the ability to adjust course as needed, balance multiple tasks and priorities such that each gets appropriate attention, and work effectively with a broad range of people.

Other Competency Models

Table 1.1 lists a number of other competency models available for healthcare leadership. The list is not exhaustive, but it does include most of the models widely used today. These models vary in focus and in methods of development, but each provides insights into effective leadership performance. Ultimately, the value of a competency model is its ability to foster more robust and meaningful conversations about performance and performance improvement.

APPLICATION TO THE C-SUITE

In many healthcare C-suites, performance is evaluated solely with operational measures, and little if any attention is paid to the executives' approach or style. As a result, some senior managers never receive meaningful feedback on their leadership competencies. Worse, practices in the C-suite set the tone for the approaches used in the rest of the organization. Initiatives in the C-suite to adopt competency models, the Nine-Box Technique, or any other standards will influence all other organizational leaders to apply more effective approaches to performance assessment and development.

Table 1.1 Healthcare Leadership Competency Models

Source(s)	Target Population	Goals	Method of Model Development	Structure
Ross, Wentzel, and Mitlyng (2002)	General (healthcare students and administrators at all levels)	Provide an in-depth treatment of competencies relevant to health administration	Author experience, review of prior models	24 competencies in 4 clusters
ACMPE (2003)	Medical group management professionals	Develop and disseminate resources to advance the development of the profession	Subject-matter expert panel and validation with incumbent sample	5 competency clusters
AUPHA (Hilberman 2004)	Graduate students and early careerists	Support pedagogy enhancement in graduate health administration education	Review of related competency models, consensus of expert panel	35 competencies in 3 clusters
Garman, Tyler, and Darnall (2004)	Early, mid-, and senior-level healthcare managers	Identify behavioral competencies that distinguish higher from lower performers	Content validation with subject-matter experts	26 competencies in 7 clusters

Table 1.1 continued

NCHL (2004)	General (healthcare management and related fields)	Develop a benchmark model of core competencies for the profession	Qualitative meta-analytic review of prior competency models (Calhoun et al. 2004); refinement based on practitioner input	26 competencies in 3 clusters
Healthcare Leadership Alliance (2005a, 2005b)	General (healthcare management at all levels)	Develop and disseminate resources for core and specialty competencies in health administration across sub-disciplines	Collaboration of five major health administration professional associations (ACHE, AONE, HFMA, HIMSS, and MGMA/ACMPE)	300 competency in 5 clusters
Dye and Garman (2006)	Senior-level executives	Support self-development in areas that differentiate the highest performers from other strong performers	Experiences of senior executive search consultants	16 competencies in 4 clusters

Note: See Garman and Johnson (2006) for the complete references for these sources.
Source: Adapted from Garman and Johnson (2006).

In contrast, leaving lower-level management to figure out and support its own methods will inevitably lead to less-effective results.[1]

If you are in the C-suite, ask yourself and your peers how talent is being defined, evaluated, and monitored within the senior management group. Most important, consider how your practices are being modeled in the organization at large.

NOTE

1. Survey research sponsored by the American College of Healthcare Executives supports this assertion. Healthcare organizations with top-down approaches to succession planning and leadership development were viewed as more effective than organizations where these activities only went on at lower leadership levels. See Garman and Tyler (2006).

REFERENCES

Dye, C., and A. N. Garman. 2006. *Exceptional Leadership: 16 Critical Competencies for Healthcare Executives.* Chicago: Health Administration Press.

———. 2008. "Real Leadership: The Advanced Course on Competencies." CEO Circle Workshop at the Annual Congress on Healthcare Leadership of the American College of Healthcare Executives, Chicago, March.

Garman, A. N., and M. Johnson. 2006, "Leadership Competencies: An Introduction." *Journal of Healthcare Management* 51 (1): 13–17.

Garman, A. N., and J. L. Tyler. 2006. *Succession Planning Practices and Outcomes in U.S. Hospital Systems: Final Report.* [Online information; retrieved 6/1/08.] www.ache.org/pubs/research/succession_planning.pdf.

CHAPTER 2

Understanding Motivation

Ciara recently completed a master's in healthcare management and is currently a fellow at Memorial Health. She meets monthly with a mentor, a well-networked executive who recommends other leaders and professionals to meet and new approaches to her work to consider. Last month, Ciara and her mentor discussed an experience that challenged her preconceived ideas about equity in organizations.

Ciara: I had always assumed that leadership levels were structured in a way that ensured superiors earned more than their direct reports. That changed after I spent several weeks with a group of first-line managers and department heads. I was amazed to learn that some of them earn less money than the people they supervise, who could take advantage of overtime and shift differentials. Many of these managers worked their way up, so I wondered why on earth anyone would take a promotion that involved a pay cut.

As I pondered that situation, I also thought about my supervisor, Lynette, with whom I feel privileged to work so closely. Although she is very busy as the CEO, putting in an 80-hour workweek, she still finds time to meet with me on a regular basis.

Mentor: You point out some insightful observations about motivation in both cases. Let's start with the line managers you met with. The currency in those positions includes many things—money, to be sure, but also autonomy and control over their schedules. Overtime is more money for a reason: The more people work, the more it interferes with their home life.

As for Lynette, she is unquestionably a great role model. This kind of devotion is not rare in the senior leadership ranks. Whether we can attribute this commitment to personal values and morals or a professional drive to serve society, we don't know for sure. You seem to be figuring out what, beyond money, motivates managers at any level to go beyond expectations. Lynette and the managers you work with are great examples of that.

Your sensitivity to people's motivation will serve you well in your career, particularly as you move into roles involving a broader set of relationships with no formal or clear lines of authority. Getting the best work out of people involves figuring out what fuels their fire and making sure you can stoke that fire.

Lynette is the first woman and minority to take the chief executive post at your hospital. She is highly focused as well. I suspect she sees a bit of herself in you, and she may be giving you all the guidance and encouragement she wished she could have received but didn't. In fact, Ciara, I think you should ask Lynette what drives her. I bet she'd give you a very thoughtful response.

As this vignette illustrates, healthcare leaders often give more than they get. Each leader's reason or motivation for his or her actions varies. As a senior executive, part of your role is to discover the unique factors that drive each of your direct reports. The more you know about the motivations of each member of your management team, the more opportunities you have to align their needs and interests with those of the organization.

In this chapter, we examine the three basic sources of motivation and their influence on leaders in general and on exceptional leaders in particular. Also, we describe the factors in the healthcare environment that either compel or repel the best executives.

SOURCES OF MOTIVATION

According to the pioneering work of David McClelland, leaders are driven by a combination of three essential needs: achievement, affiliation, and power (McClelland and Burnham 2003). These motivators are common among those in powerful positions, but the emphasis placed on each need varies from executive to executive. This emphasis, in turn, influences the leader's perceptions, behaviors, and effectiveness.

Need for Achievement

Like any other role, leadership gives an individual the opportunity to accomplish something—a task, a goal, or a vision. Leaders with a high need for achievement are particularly drawn to projects that are challenging or even riddled with problems, that have clear and quick deadlines, and that have specific and measurable goals. Executives whose driving force is achievement also consider the recognition of their accomplishments to be particularly rewarding.

Need for Affiliation

In McClelland and Burnham's typology, the need for affiliation refers to the satisfaction from being regarded favorably as a person. Although effective relationships are essential to effective leadership, leaders can be too focused on affiliation needs, to the point where being liked takes priority over accomplishing organizational goals.

Need for Power

There are two types of leadership power needs: socialized and personal. *Socialized power* involves the pursuit of influence for the good of the organization, while *personal power* involves pursuit of personal gain without regard to or even at the expense of the organization. A personal power orientation is generally counterproductive, and tolerance for it should be limited.

Fortunately, most healthcare leaders are driven less by personal power and more by socialized power, or, more familiarly, by "the need to make a difference." These executives entered the field with a calling to help others. This is especially true for administrators who started their careers as clinicians or direct caregivers. As these leaders rise into executive roles, and their power base grows, the motivator often gets fulfilled all the more deeply.

Servant leadership, a term first coined and articulated by Robert Greenleaf (2002), also describes the style of those motivated by socialized power. For servant leaders, the greatest reward is to see people benefit from their efforts. Thus, they invest time and energy in their direct reports and in their young and inexperienced protégés (as illustrated by the vignette).

Unbalanced Motivation

Your effectiveness as a leader is affected by your emphasis on these three motivators. Some executives tend to favor one over another, creating an imbalance that interferes with their decision making, development, and overall performance.

Leaders who put too much emphasis on the need for affiliation are regarded by their staff and colleagues as too soft or easily influenced. These executives struggle with any decision that involves disappointing others, and may be too willing to accommodate special requests that may go against the pursuit of organizational goals. This orientation toward wanting to be liked undermines a leader's effectiveness in serving as an agent of the organization. The higher the focus on the need for affiliation, the earlier a career can plateau.

Leaders who focus excessively on the need for achievement will be perceived as interested in *only* their own personal accomplishments. Direct reports and peers will question these executives' true motives and over time will develop mistrust. Paradoxically, these leaders may still be viewed as key contributors, outperforming colleagues in "getting the job done on time and on budget." In the face of hardship and uncertainty, however, they will find fewer supporters. A strong emphasis on the need for achievement serves entry- and mid-level managers better because these are positions in which the constant pursuit of outstanding outcomes can support the rise up the organizational ladder. At the senior level, however, this overemphasis can cause a career to stagnate.

Leaders who are strongly driven by the need for personal power (not socialized power, as described earlier) are considered by those around them as controlling. This emphasis makes a leader highly uncomfortable with not being the main decision maker or with not being able to "put his (or her) stamp" on everything. To this kind of leader, being in control feels necessary and justified because he thinks everyone else is less capable and thus needs intervention. To direct reports and other employees, this behavior discourages empowerment and undermines their contributions. As a result, the leader is not trusted, is resented for taking credit for others' work, and has a hard time building teams. Leaders who are motivated by personal power are continually faced with high staff turnover, and they often do not stay in their positions for long.

Achieving Balance: Self-Control and Adaptability

Self-control and adaptability are key qualities in balancing motivation emphasis.

According to McClelland and Burnham (2003), *self-control* (or "activity inhibition") is the hallmark of leaders with socialized (versus personal) power needs. These executives have an abundant capacity for reflective thought, allowing them to identify circumstances when their motivations or pursuits (and those of others) are not well aligned with the organization's goals. This gives these leaders the ability to see opportunities for alignment that others do not see.

Adaptability refers to the capacity to change approach when the environment changes. This trait is particularly noticeable in the event of a promotion. As noted earlier, a focus on the need for achievement can function well for employees at lower organizational levels or just beginning their careers. At this stage, staff members need to distinguish themselves through personal accomplishments to earn the attention of their supervisors and other senior leaders, who in turn may give them the chance to pursue positions of greater responsibility. Once promoted to management, however, these employees must adapt to their new status, reducing their own emphasis on achievement and replacing it with an orientation toward socialized power. Leaders at any level above a first supervisory position should spend significant time empowering their own staff. Instead of pushing their own excellence, these executives need to encourage others' success.

Effective leadership requires both self-control and adaptability. Leaders who only have self-control may be unable to change their approach even though they know doing so is the right thing to do. Leaders who are adaptive but lack self-control may change approach readily, but they may remain driven by personal motivation rather than the needs of the organization.

ORGANIZATIONAL CLIMATE AND HIGH-PERFORMING LEADERS

Leaders are attracted to some environments and are repelled by others. This section lists the organizational factors that can either pull or push great leaders.

Attractive Factors

Proximity to influence. Some positions are more influential than others, not because of their higher salaries or greater responsibilities but simply because of their placement within the organizational hierarchy. For example, numerous exceptional leaders opt to work in small organizations, and even take a pay cut, for the opportunity to report to the senior management team and to interface with the board.

When the position is not high on the organizational chart, the immediate supervisor may become an important source of influence. For example, we know of two great managers who provide their direct reports the chance to work with (and thus build relationships with) senior executives: One involves her staff in cross-departmental performance improvement projects, while the other arranges for new members of her team to meet leaders throughout the organization as an informal part of the departmental orientation process. Clearly, both leaders are aware of the development possibilities of their efforts.

Opportunity to excel. How clear and apparent are the achievement opportunities within the position and the organization? To help leaders assess this, psychologist Victor Vroom (1964) researched and articulated the "expectancy theory." According to this theory, the highest-motivating environments are those in which employees see clear linkages between (1) effort and outcomes—that is, my hard work will result in success; (2) outcomes and reward—that is, my success will be rewarded; and (3) reward and ultimate goals—that is, my rewards are well aligned with my core interests and motivators. Take, for example, a chief financial officer contemplating a new physician joint venture. She will most likely put forth considerable effort on this project if (1) she believes the project has a good chance of getting accomplished (effort–outcomes); (2) she is sure that the success of the project will yield other benefits, such as improved organizational performance or a favorable review by the board (outcomes–reward); and (3) she cares about these rewards (reward–ultimate goals).

Recognition. Good work can be recognized in several ways; however, some are particularly appealing to high-performing and career-minded leaders. For this group, *functional recognition*—acknowledgment tied explicitly to career ambitions—is the most valuable form. Ambitious leaders want to see that their outstanding work counts toward advancement opportunities. Functional recognition tells leaders whether and how they are distinguishing themselves from peers and how their achievements are positioning them for promotions.

Professional development. In this context, development refers to any activity in which a leader is building on his skills and knowledge. Strong leaders are focused not only on performing well but also on learning everything about the work itself. These executives tend to seek out and value candid feedback.

As a leader, you should take on the responsibility of ensuring that your direct reports clearly recognize the learning opportunities inherent in each new assignment. For example, if you are planning to delegate a major project to a vice president, the two of you should engage in a development-focused conversation about it beforehand. Make sure she is aware of the learning benefits of this experience, including the acquisition of new skills and knowledge and the exposure to key people with different experiences and skills. Discuss also the parts of the assignment that the vice president will be best equipped to handle or will find the most challenging. Then, during the assignment, monitor her progress and seek feedback from others involved in the work. Share their feedback and your observations with her in ways that can help her decode the lessons from the experience.

Path for advancement. A career-minded leader needs to see how his work is preparing him for future advancement, even if no specific promotion opportunity is currently available. Help your direct reports with their ambitions by providing guidance on the appropriate career pathways to pursue.

Positive organizational culture. In his book *Winning the Talent War,* Carson Dye (2002, 24–32) identified the following elements of an organizational culture that attract and retain the best leaders:

- Clear mission and vision
- Opportunities to make a difference
- Dynamic and changing environment
- Ethical operations
- Support of employee growth and learning
- Organization-wide teamwork
- Measurement and goal orientation

Repellent Factors

Excellent leaders tend to avoid the following environments.

Bureaucracy. By nature, healthcare organizations are highly bureaucratic. Bureaucracy is a necessary evil in healthcare, and eliminating it would be counterproductive, if not impossible. However, as a leader, you can do numerous things to make bureaucracy more tolerable for your leaders, including the following:

- Explain the rationale behind the bureaucracy. Why is the threshold for capital purchase review so low? Why does all travel require high-level pre-approval? Why can't budgets be set according to A instead of B? The reasons for these policies may be obvious to you, but others may only see these procedures as frustrating barriers. When you get asked why certain things are done a certain way, take the time to explain.
- Pursue better approaches with your direct reports. Many senior managers are impassioned about (or deeply disturbed by) at least one bureaucratic process. Instead of tolerating their frustrations, convince those executives to channel their strong feelings toward reconstituting the offending practice. Doing so is a productive way to both empower the leader and achieve improvements.

Dead-end positions. A post is considered dead-end if it meets more than one of the following criteria: (1) there is no clear advancement line for promotion, (2) the contribution of the job to organizational improvements is difficult or impossible to measure, or (3) it offers the job holder limited opportunities to develop new skills.

If one of your direct reports is in a dead-end position, be open and honest about his limited career trajectory within the organization, but help him develop his skills regardless of this fact. High-performing senior managers always have their careers in mind whether you talk about it or not, and if they deem that their career prospects are better elsewhere, they will leave, regardless of your counsel. What helps most in such situations is to be well informed about the leader's career plan so that you are not scrambling to fill the role because the person left unexpectedly.

APPLICATION TO THE C-SUITE

C-suite executives influence the climate that either motivates or demotivates other organizational leaders. In an ideal climate, the leaders' personal motivations are well aligned with those of the organization, and as a result, they perform well.

Here are some useful diagnostic questions to help you determine the motivational climate within your C-suite:

- How do we know if a leader (at any managerial level) is performing exceptionally? Have we established ways to communicate this information, or do we only consider this issue if the leader's superior brings it to our attention?
- How do we ensure that high performers continue to be challenged in their roles? Do we have a culture that supports job expansions and development-oriented assignments, or do we tend to focus our attention only on problem performers?
- What do we do if a leader is promotable, but an open position is not available? Do we provide development and other

opportunities instead, or do we simply hope that the leader will not leave before we can properly move her forward?

- How does our incentive and compensation system recognize excellent performance? Do high performers receive greater rewards, or do we tend to reward everyone equally?

Dissatisfied with your answers above? If so, we encourage you to develop approaches that will better engage your leaders. The human resources (HR) department may offer some strategies. However, do not overdelegate this responsibility to HR or any other department. Leaders look to your actions to set the tone for the rest of the organization.

REFERENCES

Dye, C. F. 2002. *Winning the Talent War: Ensuring Effective Leadership in Health-care*. Chicago: Health Administration Press.

Greenleaf, R. K. 2002. *Servant Leadership: A Journey into the Nature of Legitimate Power and Greatness,* 25th Anniversary Edition. Mahwah, NJ: Paulist Press.

McClelland, D. C., and D. H. Burnham. 2003. "Power Is the Great Motivator." *Harvard Business Review* 81 (1): 117–26.

Vroom, V. 1964. *Work and Motivation.* New York: Wiley.

CHAPTER 3

Navigating
Position, Career, and Life Stages

Janet is the newly appointed vice president of organizational effectiveness and leadership development. Eager for a change to work in a mission-driven organization, she left a post with a high-profile software company to return to healthcare, where she had started her career.

She spent the first few weeks on the job relearning healthcare operations, specifically those of her new employer: how the administrative and clinical pieces fit together, how leadership careers and trajectories are structured, and what motivators and challenges face management. She shadowed the leadership program offerings to find out what concepts were covered, which staff attended, and why they attended. Once she had done the preliminary work, Janet met with Linda, the system CEO, to gain Linda's perspective on the organization's needs for leadership development.

Linda: We brought you here to take our leadership development to a whole new level, to create an approach that is badly needed but has not been done in healthcare. Like a lot of healthcare systems do, we offer a full set of educational programs—manager orientations, workshops, short courses, and tuition reimbursement. It's a good, complementary collection, but unremarkable from what other systems do.

Janet: Right now you have a catalog, but what you want is a story.

Linda: You may be on to something. Say more about that.

Janet: In the past weeks, I have been studying the way leadership development is done here. As you said, we provide solid programs. But they don't add up to a compelling system.

Linda: Why do you think that is the case?

Janet: My philosophy is that for leadership development to be truly effective, it needs to be sensitive to three characteristics of each learner: position level, career stage, and life stage.

Linda: Give me some examples.

Janet: Let's take position level. Last week, I went to a leadership communication class. Most of the attendees were frontline managers, but there were also a couple of directors and one vice president. All of them needed to improve their communication skills, but effectiveness looks very different at each level. The VP needed to know how to get a consistent message delivered reliably across his division. The supervisors were looking for tips on how to deal with individual personalities.

Linda: That certainly makes sense, but I'm less clear on career and life stages.

Janet: Classes can help address immediate learning needs, but they are less helpful in addressing development across career and life stages. For these stages, we need to take a longer-term perspective. We need to adopt some practices that look beyond the classroom. I'm talking about a considerable expansion of the process, and I can make the business case for it.

Linda: What do you propose?

Janet: We need to change the paradigm from skill development to talent management, including development planning, mentoring, stretch assignments, and succession planning. The business case comes from my review of our personnel database. First, a substantial number of our senior leaders will retire at about the same time. Second, our C-suites lack diversity, and the root cause of that is we don't have diversity at lower managerial levels. We lose a disproportionate number of diverse talents and other potential leaders to other organizations. As you know, hiring from outside is both costly and risky, so we need to reach out to talented employees and give them a better chance of pursuing a long-term career here.

Linda: Development that is tailored to the individual's needs. It seems like the leadership parallel to consumer-driven care. Let me know how soon you can be ready to present a plan to the leadership council, and I'll get it on the schedule.

THE ART AND science of leadership development have changed dramatically in the past ten years. Today, many large, private organizations have established elaborate systems for continuously developing their leadership capacity. As the vignette illustrates, a recent innovative approach involves providing leadership development programs (and employee benefits) that are highly tailored to position, career, and life stages.

In this chapter, we explore the influence of position, career, and life stages on leadership development. Your awareness of these stages puts you in the best position to help others successfully navigate their development needs and align their needs with those of the organization.

No matter how driven and career-minded a leader may be, the voice of life ultimately trumps the voice of vocation. Thus, our discussion begins with life stage.

LIFE STAGE

Although every person's career pathway unfolds differently, this path is generally influenced by the three life phases: early adulthood, midlife, and post-midlife. Each phase is filled with hallmark events and challenges that have a substantial impact on how leaders regard their current and future roles.

Early Adulthood

From a career perspective, early adulthood is anchored by the first job a person takes after completing formal education. At this point, some young adults have already decided that the track to the top is the one they want to pursue. For others, the experiences in these early roles will heighten their aspirations toward leadership positions. A positive experience with a leader can inspire someone to follow in that executive's footsteps, but a negative experience may also inspire an early careerist to do better than the off-putting example. In both cases, the early-adulthood phase allows new graduates to crystallize their sense of the traits that successful leaders have, the sacrifices these leaders make, and the motivating and destructive powers of financial rewards.

Many leaders in early adulthood focus their energies on establishing their careers. They spend a substantial amount of time engaged in or thinking about work. They begin to develop habitual responses (based on what does and does not work in their jobs and relationships) for coping with stress and uncertainty. For example, they make decisions on their own, rather than ask for input, or they delegate responsibilities, rather than keep close tabs on others. Some of these mechanisms enable the leader to function well; others will need to be unlearned if they become barriers to career progress.

During early adulthood, many people enter into long-term relationships or start families. Both of these life events are almost impossible to fully plan for and can have an impact that is greater than expected, causing the need to reorder priorities. Although both male and female leaders in this phase experience the stress of life changes, women are particularly affected because they often feel pressured to make an explicit choice between career and family.

The latter part of early adulthood may be associated with promotions or greater responsibilities. With more rewards usually come additional challenges. For early adults in a two-career relationship, advancement can be a source of substantial conflict. Often one partner's job eventually takes precedence over the couple's life and requires the other partner to make major adjustments to support that person's career. Over time, this arrangement may lead to a feeling of imbalance; left unaddressed, this issue can reemerge with a vengeance at midlife.

Some leaders in the early-adult phase find that their greatest achievements happen in the workplace, not in their personal lives. These people may have difficulty developing enduring relationships outside of work, so they opt to overfocus on career accomplishments. For these leaders, the natural tendency to be in a long-term relationship or to build a family may reassert itself as early as the late 20s, in the form of feeling pressure or even panic about the prospects of remaining alone. This trepidation may lead to a sudden, goal-driven, and rapid pursuit of a mate, or it may be manifested in a yearning that is ultimately not acted on. If unresolved during early adulthood, this imbalance may also reappear during midlife.

Most people do not view the end of early adulthood as an ending; instead, it is experienced as a "settling down" period. Those in long-term relationships have reached a comfortable and predictable stage with their partners and families. Those without families have found other means of commitment and fulfillment, including friends, hobbies, and work.

Midlife

For many people, midlife involves intense introspection on the choices they have made so far in their lives. Although popular myth places midlife at or around age 40, it can begin as early as mid-30s or as late as mid-50s. Often termed a "crisis," the beginning of this phase is usually marked by either the realization of one's mortality or the reconsideration of one's life choices.

A hallmark of this phase is the reemergence of suppressed and deferred personal wants and needs, bringing along a sudden shift in priorities. For example, a leader who in the past worked long hours and showed up on the weekends may now follow a more modest work schedule. For many leaders who have reached midlife, the transformation is ultimately temporary, regardless of the intensity of the initial change. For the rest, however, the shift represents a permanent adoption of a new perspective, which could result in a change in lifestyle, location, or even vocation.

Many midlife leaders face great financial pressures, sometimes overshadowing their current or potential earnings. At this stage, those with children may be grappling with the colossal expenses of college tuition, books, and room and board. Also, their elderly parents may not be as self-sufficient, needing care that creates additional financial and time obligations. In accommodating these life changes, leaders at midlife may feel driven to find work arrangements that will allow more time flexibility, more money, or both.

Post-Midlife

Most leaders' careers extend at least ten years past the beginning of the midlife phase. Although events and challenges at post-midlife may echo those experienced at midlife, leaders at this stage usually endure more losses and grieving, including saying good-bye to former mentors and even peers. Physical decline is also clearer during this period, preventing leaders from working at the same pace and for the same length of time. Often, leaders at post-midlife begin reflecting on their career and legacy, focusing less on their own accomplishments and more on developing those who will take their place. As they approach retirement age, they should begin to disengage from the workplace to prepare for a life after retirement.

CAREER STAGE

Managing leadership career stages often involves both steady progressions and occasional shifts in approach. In their book on leadership transitions, Charan, Drotter, and Noel (2001) present a "pipeline" model in which the pathway up the career ladder is bent at key junctures. Psychologist Arthur Freedman (1998) offers a similar model that uses "crossroads." The crossroads represent the fundamental shift a leader needs to make in her approach when ascending to a new career stage. More than refining existing skills, these crossroads demand a different approach to the work itself. As depicted in Figure 3.1, at least four career stages in healthcare leadership require such a shift.

Influencer

We have termed the first career stage *influencer*. In this role, a person's success depends on coordinating the efforts of people who do not report to her. Examples include planning analysts and quality coordinators, both of whom need accurate and timely data from various departments to do their work. When navigated successfully, the influencer stage teaches the person how to move others toward achieving a goal without relying on formal authority. This critical lesson, along with many others, can be carried forward to the next career stage, when the person becomes a formal leader with a set of direct reports. At the next stage, the leader can continue to exert influence rather than authority, and in doing so engender an environment in which employees are empowered.

Manager

We define the manager career stage by responsibility, not title. The stage begins the first time that a person has administrative authority over direct reports. At this point, the leader must shift his orientation away from doing all the work himself and toward delegating the work to others, and from being responsible only for his own performance to being ultimately accountable for his staff's quality of work. Also, the leader needs to learn to cede control,

Figure 3.1 Position Stages and Crossroads at the Four Leadership Career Stages

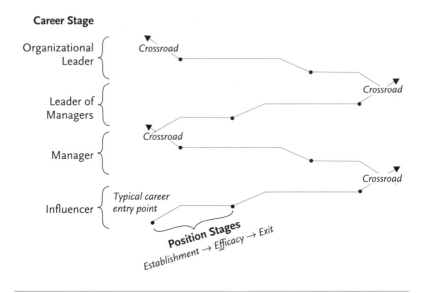

enabling his direct reports the latitude to own their projects and assignments. However, the leader must establish acceptable levels of performance so that he knows the limits of underperformance and can appropriately address these problems when they come up.

In addition to these new human resource challenges, management positions often involve a substantial increase in job complexity across a number of fronts. Thus, leaders at the manager level may need to equip themselves with a sophisticated understanding of health law, finance, quality improvement, marketing, and other management-related areas. Beyond their own learning, manager-level leaders will benefit from developing working relationships with other leaders who have more experience or expertise in these areas. These people can serve as just-in-time resources when unfamiliar problems arise.

Leader of Managers

At this stage, the leader is in charge of a team of managers. In many organizations, this position carries a vice president title. The nature of the work at this level is threefold—managerial, operational, and strategic. From the managerial perspective, the leader is using her hands-on knowledge of the demands and challenges of the front line to provide guidance and to develop the skills of her team members, enabling them to manage with autonomy. From the operations perspective, the leader is thinking in terms of how her department's metrics are set and how her managers are performing against these metrics. From the strategy perspective, she is looking at ways in which the functions, needs, challenges, and goals of her various areas fit into the strategies of the broader organization, and at how the areas or departments will need to evolve over time to remain in step.

Leaders of managers need to develop a more elaborate mental model of the organization, one that recognizes the competing priorities and trade-offs other departments represent to the organizational leaders. This broader understanding allows leaders of managers to better advocate for resources and to better find promising opportunities for collaboration and mutual assistance with colleagues at their level. Forming relationships with peers is particularly important at this stage, not only for the purpose of getting the task at hand done but also for cultivating a base of supporters for later career pursuits.

Organizational Leader

The final career stage requires the leader to have a comprehensive understanding of the context in which the organization operates. As such, an organizational leader devotes a lot of time and energy to working with the board or the community and being the face or spokesperson of the institution.

At this level, the leader's development focus shifts from the individual to the culture. Here, the leader should be providing continuous learning and advancement to his direct reports to set an example, fostering an organizational climate that values the development of all employees. Also, at this stage, the need for effective mass communication becomes more pronounced, so the leader must learn new ways to disseminate information across many organizational layers.

Retirement

Most leaders experience retirement not as an endpoint but as another career stage. Many such leaders, particularly those who were highly invested in their careers, find the transition from organizational leader to retired leader extremely difficult. Advance preparation is helpful, allowing retirees to carefully plan not only what they want to do to fill up newfound time but also how they can continue to meet their powerful motivational needs.

With a little advanced planning, many retired leaders thrive in a rewarding post-executive world, which may involve teaching, volunteer work, and/or executive-in-residence posts. The key for leaders at this final career stage is to explore their many options ahead of time. Coming up with a satisfactory plan at the last minute almost never worked during their leadership tenure and will not work at their retirement stage.

POSITION STAGE

Leaders typically move through at least one position at each career stage. Within each position are at least three distinct stages that we have termed *establishment, efficacy,* and *exit.* These stages are illustrated graphically in Figure 3.1, as a bracket under one of the positions in the "influencer" career stage.

Establishment

The focus of the establishment stage is learning about the position: What the role entails, what working relationships need to be developed, and how success will be defined are just some of the common questions answered during this stage. The amount of time a leader spends in this stage depends on the complexity of the job, the type of relationship (collegial, detached, or hostile) he has with his direct supervisor, and his capacity to learn.

According to our observations, this period typically lasts a year or longer, but it is almost never shorter than three or four months. During establishment, the leader listens more than acts and leans heavily on the supervisor for direction and insight. A leader who fails to receive supervisor attention, support, and guidance may feel pressured to perform "at all costs," which will interfere with the leader's ability to learn.

Efficacy

In the efficacy phase, the leader, who is now well equipped with foundational knowledge and has successfully completed some projects, turns her attention to pursuing and maintaining performance gains in the areas for which she is responsible. The length of this stage varies, depending on the leader's career interest, trajectory, and available promotion options. Note that career-minded and ambitious leaders may set a goal for how long they stay in this stage for a given position; that period could be as short as one year but is rarely longer than three years.

Exit

The exit stage begins when the leader decides he is ready to move on from the position. The briefest of the three position stages, exit can be as short as a few months. Longer exit periods are better for smoother transitions but are only possible if a leader and his direct report discuss these transitions openly. Leaders whose performance and actions are under close scrutiny, or who fear retaliation for talking honestly about their ambitions or position dissatisfaction, may have shorter exit phases and may leave their organizations with less of a transition plan. Exceptional leaders more carefully plan their exit, identifying and developing potential successors and signaling (if not outright communicating) their intention to depart at least six months ahead of time.

Post-exit, the leader will begin his new position at the establishment phase, and the cycle will repeat itself for the new role.

APPLICATION TO THE C-SUITE

In many healthcare organizations, a gap between the C-suite and the level below it is created by differences in both career and life stages. For example, a CEO who is near retirement may oversee executives in early or midlife phase. Other members of senior management may have reached their career goals but may be in charge of leaders who are still aggressively pursuing theirs. The breadth of stages may cause internal resentments and conflicting viewpoints and approaches, but this situation is an unavoidable part of organizational dynamics.

As a chief leader, you should understand how the different stages your team members are experiencing affect their work behavior, mind-set, and decision making. This familiarity will also enable you to support their career progression and plans, whether those paths involve staying in place or leaving.

REFERENCES

Charan, R., S. Drotter, and J. Noel. 2001. *The Leadership Pipeline: How to Build the Leadership-Powered Company.* San Francisco: Jossey-Bass.

Freedman, A. M. 1998. "Pathways and Crossroads to Institutional Leadership." *Consulting Psychology Journal: Practice & Research* 50 (3): 131–51.

CHAPTER 4

Learning by Leading

Judith is a partner in a leadership development consulting firm, and she was recently nominated to serve on the national board of a large healthcare system. At the end of the two-day board orientation, she was approached by Sister Mary, the CEO of the organization.

Sister Mary: Once you get acclimated, I would like to hear your ideas about our leadership development and succession planning efforts. Perhaps you may be interested in leading the board's human resources committee.

Judith: I have had informal discussions about this with some members of senior management and the board. I see opportunities to make improvements here.

Sister Mary: Splendid! Tell me your initial thoughts.

Judith: The work this system has put in to develop the Leadership University is impressive. However, we need to be careful about how we define its success.

Sister Mary: What do you mean?

Judith: In the 1980s and '90s, a lot of *Fortune* 500 companies devised their own corporate universities. These programs got so big and mismanaged that their original intent was lost. As a result, the organizations began equating the length of their course catalogs to their excellence—the more classes they offered, the better they thought they were doing. Some didn't even bother to collect data from learners. If they did, it was to document how well these attendees enjoyed the session rather than how it affected their performance. Moreover, recent studies have shown that most leadership growth is the result of experiences rather than classroom lessons. Workshops and courses are important, but they must be supplemented with opportunities to put theory into practice; otherwise, performance cannot improve much. I suggest we move away from the idea of leadership development as an event that people attend. Instead, we should think of it as a fundamental part of the work itself. For example, the Leadership University could have a non-classroom structure that promotes on-the-job learning. We should develop a core competency for helping senior leaders create cross-training programs and stretch assignments.

Sister Mary: You made insightful points. On the one hand, I agree that we should invest a lot in our people. On the other, I'm not convinced that we get the most 'mission for our money' if we spend a small fortune to sponsor workshops and short courses that may not yield the results we're after.

Judith: Some of these courses are worth retaining, but we need to monitor them carefully to determine which ones. The same will be true for the work-based learning. In my role on the board, I want to make sure your leadership investments are made as wisely as possible.

AS THIS VIGNETTE expresses, leadership development is most efficient and effective when given on the job about the job. In this chapter, we describe how leaders learn from experience and how you can help this process along.

LEARNING IN THE WORKPLACE

Leadership is a vocation learned primarily on the job. Leaders' skills develop most rapidly in response to the environmental demands placed on them, because these are the areas where they get the most practice and feedback. Even the most successful classroom-based leadership training programs are designed to improve job-specific outcomes and processes. Learning that is not relevant to the actual expectations and practice of the job is rarely, if at all, applied and almost never improves performance.

Success and speed of workplace learning are heavily influenced by the learner's (1) awareness of his learning needs, (2) work experiences, and (3) learning orientation.

AWARENESS OF LEARNING NEEDS

Consider this story: After ten years in his current position, a senior manager is looking for a new job. He meets with a recruiter who asks him to describe the nature of his work and the lessons he learned over the years. The senior manager responds by listing the tasks he does in his role: budgeting, staffing, negotiating contracts, and so on. He mentions that he completes these tasks year in and year out, and these responsibilities have stayed constant during his tenure in the organization. Also, he states that his superior is "hands-off" and thereby allows him a great deal of autonomy. The recruiter ponders his answer then says, "It sounds like you really don't have ten years of experience. It sounds like you have one year of experience that you repeated ten times."

Is the recruiter being unfair? Maybe. But is the recruiter being honest? Definitely.

The basic message of this anecdote is this: Expertise is not a product of experience alone. Feedback from other people is also essential. The senior manager in this story received little feedback from his boss, colleagues, direct reports, and other work associates. As a result, his career is stagnating, although he seems to think he has mastered the role. Self-assessment by itself is not sufficient; often, it perpetuates biased views rather than corrects them.

Blind Spots of Self-Assessment

Throughout the course of our work, we continually self-assess, identifying the areas in which we think we excel and those in which we think we need to improve. As compelling as our judgments can feel, they are merely perception, not reality. The confidence we feel in our self-assessments is actually an outright self-deception.[1]

The truth is, our brains are not well designed for accurate self-evaluation. Fortunately, many of us can assess others' actions just fine. What this means is that the only reliable way to assess your capability and potential is to ask the people you work with—and the ones whose judgment you trust.

Four-Quadrant Model

Most of what we do on the job is intuitive—that is, we are told what to do, we do it, and we find out the result of our effort later. The more we do a particular activity, the less we think about how to do it. Eventually, the activity becomes almost automatic.

Leadership learning, however, requires more active and conscious participation. Figure 4.1 illustrates the four quadrants of learning;[2] each of these quadrants indicates the learner's self-awareness and performance capability. Understanding how these quadrants fit together allows you to determine a leader's learning needs.

In Quadrant I: Unconscious Development Need, a leader does not know that she is either lacking or deficient in a competency area. Before she can improve in a specific area, she must first learn about her shortcoming from those who observe or supervise her performance. Employee surveys, 360-degree assessment, and direct feedback all can reveal improvement and learning needs. Quadrant II: Conscious Development Need is the next phase, wherein the leader is aware of his development need and thus can attend to it appropriately. Over time, the leader will gain a more sophisticated and comprehensive understanding of the area in which he is lacking and will be apt to pursue improvement through practice and feedback.

Continued practice and feedback are the hallmark of Quadrant III: Conscious Proficiency. Here, the leader's mindfulness results in

Figure 4.1 Four Quadrants of Learning

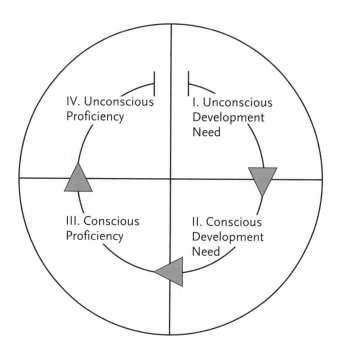

better performance and more consistently positive feedback from others. The final phase is Quadrant IV: Unconscious Proficiency. At this point, the leader has mastered the skill to the point where she can consistently deliver an outstanding performance without putting conscious effort into it.

In some competencies, some leaders go through Quadrant I through Quadrant IV quickly, while others slowly advance from one phase to the next. This length of time is influenced by many variables, only some of which are under the leader's direct control. The three factors that have the greatest influence on pace of learning are (1) availability of practice opportunities, (2) availability of high-quality feedback on performance, and (3) the leader's capacity for learning.

TYPES OF WORK EXPERIENCES

The learning value of a given work experience varies depending on several factors. For example, an ideal work experience is demanding and novel enough to compel a leader to focus and to try new approaches. However, the experience cannot be so demanding and novel that the risk of failure is high and the leader feels lost. A research review by McCauley and Brutus (1998) identified four types of work experiences that are particularly valuable for on-the-job learning.

Unfamiliar Responsibilities

Tasks or roles that require new responsibilities tend to be associated with rapid learning. New demands disrupt old routines, causing the leader to pay attention to (or even rethink) existing assumptions and approaches. "Unfamiliar territory" also spurs the leader to look for guides or mentors who know or have experience with the terrain. Having a guide can enhance and speed up the learning process.

Need for Substantial Change

Assignments or roles that demand implementation of change also usher in learning. In this case, existing assumptions and relationships are examined, challenged, and altered. This close scrutiny helps the leader establish a strategy for pursuing change.

A change initiative often requires the development of new relationships built on trust. Trusted allies become additional sources of feedback, providing the leader with honest and straightforward critiques of his performance and improvement needs.

Greater Responsibility or Latitude

Expansion of responsibility entails an increase in areas of accountability—new budgets, staff, services, or outcomes, for example. In contrast, expansion of latitude involves growth in power but may not mean more responsibilities—new authority over purchases or new ability to make executive decisions about policies and programs, for example.

Expansion in either responsibility or latitude heightens learning for several reasons. First, it gives the leader more opportunities to work with, and thus understand, the broader organizational system. Second, it draws the leader's conscious attention to processes and outcomes. Third, it enables the leader to experiment with more options, solutions, and approaches.

Dealing with Failure or Adversity

The work experience of failure and adversity almost always delivers valuable learning. A *failure* can be defined as falling short of expected outcomes. Common examples of failure include a widely missed target or substantial decline in market share, and demotions or terminations. *Adversity* can be defined as substantial environmental barriers to success. Common examples of adversity include unexpected/unfavorable changes in policies or regulations, a hostile relationship with an influential physician or another executive, and lack of organizational support for one's programs.

Failure and adversity rarely seem to be useful learning experiences at that moment. Turning these hardships into lessons requires mental reframing. That is, when adequate time has passed and the matter has been resolved, the leader should reflect on the experience and mine it for insight. For example, the experience of being passed over for a promotion may reveal a character trait or skill deficiency that had been overlooked or pushed aside. Recognizing this shortfall is an essential first step in improving.

LEARNING ORIENTATION

The third factor that influences learning on the job is a person's inclination toward learning itself. Leaders differ in their capacity to learn from experiences. However, research by McCauley (2001) revealed that high-performing leaders share a common trait: They see the learning potential in all aspects of their work. They leverage this orientation further by seeking out their colleagues' feedback to continually identify and pursue opportunities to improve their skills and knowledge.

These highly successful leaders also have in common the following learning characteristics:

- *Proactive approach to challenges.* This trait is marked by an intrepid resolve to take responsibility and control in the face of ambiguity and adversity. Young leaders with this approach get noticed more quickly by their superiors and thus receive more rapid promotions.
- *Habit of critical reflection.* Exceptional leaders continually challenge fundamental assumptions: Why do we do things a certain way? What other options do we have? How can we do this even better next time? Often inwardly directed, these questions allow the leader to examine current practices and perspectives, identify mistakes and corrections, and pursue alternatives.
- *Openness to new approaches and perspectives.* This characteristic drives excellent leaders to carefully consider various and differing opinions and methods. They are less likely to quickly

dismiss people's suggestions and more likely to try them to find out if they will yield improvements. Such openness to possibilities presents these leaders with more opportunities for learning and experiences.

APPLICATION TO THE C-SUITE

Opportunities for on-the-job development and learning become more valuable (but more difficult to provide and manage) at higher leadership levels. Thus, C-suite executives must encourage and assist their managers and directors to move in and out of positions and functional areas so that they can get broader experience. For example, the chief financial officer may assign a finance manager to work in the strategic marketing and communications department for a year. This type of immersion will expose the finance manager to different parts of the organization and will allow her a richer appreciation for how these departments run. Many vice presidents are too protective of their leaders. As a consequence, the leaders do not develop an understanding of other areas in the organization. In many industries, managerial job rotation is an important element of succession planning and talent management.

In addition, C-suite executives must employ and strengthen their organization's performance feedback systems. As discussed in this chapter, an environment rich in feedback enables learning and improvement.

NOTES

1. For research on self-perception, see Wilson and Dunn (2004).

2. This four-quadrant model is widely used by leadership educators, and we were unable to trace its point of origin. For an expanded description of this model, see Whitmore (1996).

REFERENCES

McCauley, C. D. 2001. "Leader Training and Development." In *The Nature of Organizational Leadership: Understanding the Performance Imperatives Confronting Today's Leaders,* edited by S. J. Zaccaro and R. J. Klimoski. San Francisco: Jossey-Bass.

McCauley, C. D., and S. Brutus. 1998. *Management Through Job Experiences: An Annotated Bibliography.* Greensboro, NC: Center for Creative Leadership.

Whitmore, J. 1996. *Coaching for Performance: The New Education of the Practical Guide.* Sonoma, CA: Nicholas Brealey Publishing.

Wilson, T. D., and E. W. Dunn. 2004. "Self-Knowledge: Its Limits, Value, and Potential for Improvement." *Annual Review of Psychology* 55: 493–518.

PART II

CHAPTER 5

Conducting a
Developmental Interview

Paula is the new administrative fellow at the flagship hospital of a healthcare delivery system. In the last several months, she has completed projects for various leaders throughout the facility. In the hospital, the process for matching fellows with projects is highly informal: An executive identifies a need and then describes that need to the fellow, who then carries out the task. Word has gotten out that Paula is particularly talented and that her skills are in high demand. Currently, she is meeting with Dennis, the chief information officer, to decide if his department and its needs are a good fit for her development.

Dennis: Thanks for coming by so early in the morning, Paula. I've heard great things about you, and I'm eager to convince you that you ought to work with me.

Paula: I appreciate your sending me a briefing in advance. It gives me a better understanding of the IT department's needs. Selecting to work here would allow me to learn more about workflow, clinician relations, and electronic medical records. From that perspective, this opportunity seems a great fit. Before I agree to the assignment though, I need reassurance on a few things.

Dennis: I'm all ears.

Paula: First, I suspect that accessing the clinicians will be the toughest part of this assignment. So I need guidance from someone who has experience and knowledge in working with doctors. This person has to come when I facilitate meetings with clinicians so that we can debrief afterward about my performance.

Dennis: Dr. Schultz is our clinical liaison. He does attend most of our meetings, but he is a busy man. I can't guarantee that he can stay afterward to give you feedback. I will talk to him about this and let you know his decision.

Paula: I'll wait for his response. My next request concerns getting feedback on my style. I've been told that I can be pushy. Although I am really focused on delivering successful projects, I don't want to alienate people in the process. A mentor will be able to help me improve the way I come across.

Dennis: I can do that for you.

Paula: Great! The other part of this feedback involves your staff. Into my third or fourth month, I'd like you to ask at least five of your employees to evaluate not just my working style but also my progress on the project. I'll provide you with a specific description of the competencies I'd like evaluated and a survey form. All you have to do is to encourage staff to participate.

Dennis: That's very doable.

Paula: Terrific. I'll look forward to working with you once you let me know that Dr. Schultz is on board.

Dennis: Wonderful! Even in our short conversation, I can see how you have earned your reputation. I'm very impressed with the thought and planning you put into developing your skills.

Paula: I have the first mentor on my first rotation to thank for that. She did a developmental interview with me, which I have been using to guide me ever since.

THIS VIGNETTE MAY seem too good to be true in the real world. After all, how often do we see nascent leaders take such a sophisticated and structured approach to their own development? In this chapter, we offer a framework for establishing a development plan (similar to the one Paula follows) that is comprehensive but does not require a lot of time to implement and monitor. Called Developmental Interview (DI), this process is particularly well suited for new hires or recently promoted leaders.

In a nutshell, the DI is a data-collection and analysis tool that you and your direct reports or protégés may use to reach a shared understanding of their career goals, the job's required competencies (skills, knowledge, and abilities), the competency areas in which they need improvement, and the development plan of action. An example of the DI Guide—the actual document to be filled out—is provided in Appendix A at the end of this book.

GUIDELINES FOR INTRODUCING THE PROCESS

Although there is no right or wrong way to implement a DI, there is a recommended approach (based on our experience) that will ease you and your direct reports into the DI method.

Time Frame

Conduct the DI "off cycle" from the scheduled performance appraisal. For example, if the performance appraisal is in August, then defer the DI until February. The reason these two processes should be separated is to ensure that the DI is viewed as a development, rather than an appraisal, activity.

Advance Work

The first three sections of the DI Guide contain questions that may be challenging to answer thoughtfully. Accurate and honest responses to these questions are critical. Thus, we recommend that you ask your direct report to think about these questions before the actual interview. By giving this person the benefit of advance notice, you are enabling her to reflect on her current and future career demands. Even if initially the person only provides top-of-mind answers, she has started the process of thinking. At the actual interview, allow the person to further clarify and evolve her thoughts.

Initial Inquiries

Expect your direct report to ask questions about the DI process and the DI Guide itself. Following are some common queries, along with our suggested answers.

- *Why do I need to complete a DI?* This process leads us to an in-depth discussion about your career interests and goals and what we both can do to move toward those goals. The attention we pay to your career can benefit you now and in the future.
- *Some of the questions on the Guide are sensitive. How honest should my answers be?* Some questions, such as how long do you plan to stay in your position and with the organization, may seem strange to discuss directly with your boss. However, if you can openly discuss these issues with me, I will be better equipped to support you in your career goals. If you are still concerned about talking openly about these questions, I'd like you to help me understand how you think the conversation could harm you, so we can overcome these hesitations.
- *How will the DI affect my performance review?* My hope is that this process will help you achieve your current and future performance review goals. But the DI is different from the assessment process. We are not evaluating your work to determine whether or not you reached the established performance goals. We are doing this to plan how you can improve and build on your existing capabilities in ways that will support your job and career.
- *A lot of these questions deal with the future. What if my answers change over time?* I will not consider your responses to be set in stone. Development means evolution, and I expect that your thoughts about your career path will change as you progress professionally. This DI process is only the start to that ongoing dialogue.

THE DI MEETING

When the DI Guide has been completed, a face-to-face meeting should be scheduled. In this meeting, you and your direct report should discuss each item in the Guide. This is the time to ask and answer additional questions, to clarify responses, and to expound on ideas. To help you navigate each section in the Guide during this meeting, we recommend the following approach.

Section One: Position and Career Goals

Section One is designed to get the interviewee thinking about being in his position for a finite period of time, in preparation for the next phase of his career.

Ideally, how long would you like to remain in this role? The length of time given here indicates the person's mental model regarding the progress of his career. Depending on the person's degree of ambition or drive, this time may seem too short, too long, or just right to you. If the time frame is realistic, say so. If not, find out the reasoning behind the response. For example, if the time seems excessively long (e.g., ten years), you may explain that the typical length of service in such a role is five years or less because after a few years, the position leads to greater opportunities. Regardless of the response to this question, it is valuable to ask how the person reached his answer.

What in your current role is working particularly well? The answer to this question can reveal several important things. In addition to giving you the interviewee's self-assessment, it can tell you what she is most proud of and, by extension, what is most important to her. This can also be used as a jumping-off point for encouraging her to pursue development in areas in which she may be weak. For example, to an interviewee who shines in budgeting, you may say, "Your public speaking skills can be improved to the degree that they can be considered as much of an asset as your budgeting skills."

The other consideration here is how others' opinions informed the person's response. You may ask if she approached her peers or tapped into their previous feedback on her strengths and accomplishments. (Failure to use feedback may itself suggest a skill-development need.) Some sample questions to pose include, What led you to select this area? Have you always seen this area as a strength? Why do you think this area works well?

What are you finding the most challenging in your current role? The contrast between the "most challenging" and the "particularly well" questions is useful to consider. Often, people attribute successes to things they can control, and problems to factors they deem to be beyond their control. Here, the person may assign blame for his frustration and challenges to an individual, a department, or a resource constraint. In such a case, you can intervene. Help him to recognize the aspects that he can control and thus change and to identify new approaches.

Useful follow-up questions include, What led you to select this area as most challenging? Have you experienced a similar conflict before? What solutions have you applied? How is this challenge affecting you as an individual?

If your current role could be made ideal, in what ways would it be different from how it is currently? The answer offers an insight into what can motivate the person to develop. To expand this question, you may ask, What strategies have you tried so far to bring about improvement?

Future position(s). These questions are designed to yield insights for motivating development. The longer-term focus serves as a vehicle for career coaching, enabling you to suggest additional perspectives and pathways that the person was not aware of before.

Career and organizational setting. This part of the DI Guide concerns job mobility. Most employees, regardless of position level, will not discuss with their immediate supervisors their plans to leave when a better opportunity comes, simply because they do not want to be viewed as disloyal or incur any job-related consequences. Conversely, many superiors are reluctant to bring up the topic, lest they "put the idea" in their direct reports' heads.

This conversation is considered taboo by many professionals. However, we argue that such a conversation is critical, given that in the United States, the concept of growing up in and retiring from a single organization has become the exception rather than the rule. In healthcare, particularly, job mobility (both for position and location purposes) is not unusual.

Your career-minded direct report will contemplate career moves on her own, whether or not you initiate a conversation about it. By providing a forum for an open dialogue, you are orchestrating a smooth transition, enabling you both to be prepared for the inevitable. If your direct report is uneasy or hesitant about this topic, sometimes sharing your own or others' positive experiences in moving from one organization to the next can help her gain comfort that the subject is not as dangerous as it may seem.

Section Two: Career History and Experiences with Leadership Development

Section Two relates to the path the person has taken to develop his competencies thus far. The responses here identify development methods that have worked well, which will in turn guide both of you to determine the most ideal path for the future.

In reviewing this section, ask the person to expand his answers with questions like these:

- Walk me through your first growth opportunity or promotion. What did you learn?

- How did you receive feedback? Who gave it to you, and what approach did they use?
- What about your previous development experiences have made them successful?

After this review, explore the common themes that arose with follow-up questions such as, What patterns do you see here in terms of the methods that match well with your learning style and interests? and To avoid our use of ineffective approaches, tell me about the unfavorable development experiences you have had.

Section Three: Current and Future Competency Development Needs

The focus of Section Three is on the actual feedback and experience, as opposed to self-assessment (which is often inaccurate), regarding strengths and weaknesses.

In this section, you should examine each item and not favor only the parts that deal directly with development needs. Discussing each area ensures that you have a complete understanding of the person's experiences and allows her to articulate her grasp of each competency. (Conversely, selecting certain parts for discussion will send the message that the other areas are not important and thus deserve little or no attention.) Most importantly, however, a full exploration of this section will reveal the person's blind spots—that is, the areas that she is unaware need to be developed, or Quadrant I in the learning matrix from Chapter 4.

You can bring these blind spots into the light by defining the competency in question and by bringing up recent events. For example, "I have noticed an improvement opportunity in listening—specifically, letting people finish their thoughts rather than talking over them. This can be tough to do in executive committee meetings when opinions are so strong and the schedule is so tight, so it's a particularly good place to get practice." Also, you may remind her of specific feedback you have given her in the past, such as, "Last year, we talked about the need to develop a more compelling vision for your department. What can we do to move us toward that goal?"

The summary portion of Section Three allows you to reassess the development priorities according to the discussion you just had. For example, if the person initially rated listening as "most developed," but after your exploration it is revealed as "most in need of improvement," then its place on the priority list should be pushed up. During this process, however, be mindful not to overpower your direct report. Be gentle and tactful, giving consideration to his career aspirations at the same time: "All of the areas you have selected for improvement are right on target. We have discussed other areas that also need attention, so I suggest we add those as well. You only have so much time to devote to development, so let's make sure we are prioritizing appropriately. We can take the less urgent ones off the list, then add them on as the others are accomplished. Does that sound reasonable?"

Section Four: Development Plan

The eight questions in this section lead to the creation of a well-structured development plan complete with a timeline, articulated goals, and monitoring and feedback systems. The sample DI Guide in Appendix A provides two options for setting up such a plan—project/assignment-based and competency-based.

We generally recommend the project/assignment-based option, given that most learning takes place within the context of work experience (as discussed in Chapter 4). However, a competency-based approach makes sense in a situation where the leader is weak in a certain competency area or has to learn a specific skill set. Areas in which the competency-based option is effective include public speaking, business writing, and strategic planning. In these cases, the leader may attend courses and workshops or may participate in activities that enhance these skills; these activities can be external and may not necessarily link to internal projects or assignments.

The project/assignment-based alternative revolves around in-house initiatives that provide growth opportunities. We recommend that the total number of such projects not exceed two or three at one time. Limiting this number helps ensure that each assignment is properly monitored and followed up and receives adequate time and attention. Chapter 4 provides guidance about which kinds of assignments yield the greatest learning value. Following are our recommendations for documenting these assignments in a development plan.

Project/assignment title. Give each project/assignment a short, descriptive name—for example, "Service Standards." This brief title provides an easy reference for future discussion.

Description. Be brief, clear, and to the point. Provide a short description of the project to be undertaken, the outcomes to be achieved, and the approaches to be used.

Goals. Describe clearly what the project will accomplish for the organization and the interviewee. If the assignment is a training program, explain the learning objectives that are expected and the areas where they will be applied.

Contacts/sponsors. Identify people who can provide support and information, especially if the project involves other departments, organizations, and stakeholders. These individuals can also serve as additional sources of feedback for the leader.

Skills/competencies for development. List the skills that the assignment will require the person to learn, practice, or improve. Select the competencies that are most important for him to develop, then monitor his progress throughout the assignment. This identified set of skills can also serve as the focus of feedback at the completion of the project.

From whom will feedback be collected on development? The key word in this question is "will," not "might" or "could." Determine the appropriate individuals who will commit to providing input on the person's work. Part b of this question delves into the finer detail of the feedback-collection process, including who is accountable for asking for feedback, especially when it is not delivered face-to-face.

Development resources. Encourage your direct report to check out books, articles, and workshops and to seek out a mentor—all of which will contribute to her development as she undertakes the assignment. You can also point her to resources that will match her preferred approach to learning.

Check-in. Note the dates or milestones when you expect to check on the leader's progress. We recommend that you "hardwire" these dates into your electronic or paper calendar. If schedules and priorities change later, reset the appointment or tack it on to the agenda of a standing meeting with this leader. At these follow-ups, discuss the elements that either impede or speed his momentum and offer advice if needed.

Generally, checking in should be the direct report's responsibility, as it indicates the level of his commitment to this process. However, you also should track the dates of these progress conversations to ensure that they happen. Busyness is a convenient excuse for avoiding a follow-up, so the monitoring responsibility is best shared.

APPLICATION TO THE C-SUITE

For C-suite executives, the time required to initiate the DI process can become a barrier to implementing this useful approach to leadership development. If you fit in this category, consider delegating the initial DI work (not the actual development nor monitoring/ feedback) to another professional, either internal or external, who has experience in senior-level development. An executive coach with experience in the healthcare setting is also a good alternative. After the development plan is established, however, you still need to provide regular monitoring and feedback. This step will require consistency but not as much time investment.

As a chief leader, your attitude and perspective about leadership development are constantly being watched and adopted by your staff. As such, we strongly recommend that you role-model a positive approach to developing your own competencies. We provide guidance on modeling a positive developmental climate in Figure 5.1.

Figure 5.1 Modeling a Positive Development Climate

The most powerful approach to engendering a culture of career development and growth is to demonstrate your commitment to your own development.

- *Provide a balanced description.* Discussing your strengths is not enough. You also have to declare the areas you are working to improve. Doing so sends the message that we all have development needs to work on.
- *Be unapologetic.* Acknowledge your shortcomings, but do not apologize for them. Not apologizing underscores that development is a normal and important part of leadership.
- *Invite feedback.* Encourage those who work with you to provide input for your development. This practice models good feedback-seeking habits for your direct reports and mentees.
- *Express optimism.* Share your past failures and accomplishments. Your direct reports will appreciate learning that you have pursued and continue to pursue improvement and growth opportunities.

CHAPTER 6

Sustaining a Development Focus

Carol, the vice president of human resources in a not-for-profit hospital, is in charge of the organization's leadership development programs. Her work was instrumental in the formation of the institution's leadership competency model. Her next step is to make a presentation to the board's human resource committee to propose a plan for using the model to support hiring and development. To prepare for the meeting, Carol decides to approach Dr. Cieslak, the chief medical officer, to ask him to review her presentation and to get a sense of his perspective in advance.

Dr. Cieslak: I see where you're going with this proposal, and the medical staff can certainly use more development attention. I am unclear, though, on the notion that each job level has its own corresponding competencies. What happens when a staff member is performing at a higher level than the competencies associated with his job? Surely, I can't just give him a new title.

Carol: Right. An employee's title describes his current responsibilities—the job he is doing, not the job he is capable of. A lot of this work is about developing talent in anticipation of future need. We want people to be preparing in advance for potential future promotions. To do that, they need to know what kinds of competencies are involved with the next level of leadership, and they need to work on them ahead of time.

Dr. Cieslak: I need to better understand how this will support our core mission, which is to provide safe, high-quality care. Can I assume you have hard data to back that up?

Carol: Rest assured, we are taking an evidence-based approach. Our competency model will tie to a set of practices with clear research support: personnel selection, training, employee engagement, and the like.

Dr. Cieslak: Where are you finding this evidence? I haven't seen anything about it in any of the journals I read.

Carol: Much of the research on human resources practices, including use of competency models, is published outside of healthcare. You have to look in the management journals. I can provide you with copies of these studies, if you like.

Dr. Cieslak: I'm glad you're ready to answer that question, and you should expect it from the board. My last fundamental concern about leadership development is this: We try our best to recruit and retain only the best employees and doctors. With leadership development, we are showing our care for people's professional growth. But in a small organization like ours, the number of available leadership positions is limited. Two of my associates have left for another organization because we could not offer them a promotion. With due respect to the intent of your initiative, aren't we just accelerating the process of pushing people out the door by putting so much emphasis on preparing them to be leaders?

THIS VIGNETTE DEMONSTRATES several common difficulties experienced when initiating leadership development efforts in healthcare organizations. Here, the conflict goes beyond limited time and resources. Often, these initiatives reveal basic differences in whether and how leaders see potential benefits and the risks of developing their staff. These differences are important to surface and discuss, and they should not become perpetual excuses to delay moving forward.

This book supports the contention that leadership development must be viewed as a long-term investment strategy. There is a start-up cost in the form of identifying needs, allocating time, and adjusting habit/behavior for addressing these needs. This investment portfolio then must be watched regularly. There will be some small, quick payoffs and, ultimately, more substantial, long-term payoffs.

In this chapter, we propose strategies for assessing your own development attitude and practice and for supporting development through proactive, efficient, and regular feedback. We also present the common reasons that development is not considered a priority in many organizations.

TRANSFORMING YOUR DEVELOPMENT MIND-SET

Ask yourself, "During a typical week, how much time do I spend giving my direct reports feedback?" According to the Economist Intelligence Unit (2006), senior executives at organizations that have a stellar reputation for developing their staff devote as much as 20 percent of their time to development activities. This same study suggests that at least 5 percent (or several hours per week) of a senior manager's time should be invested in developing staff. But how do executives pull this off and keep it going? The answer is that most leaders find a return on their time in the form of higher-performing direct reports. In other words, development work will free up your schedule, because as your staff obtain, improve, and master skills you will be able to delegate more work.

In Chapter 5, we laid out the process for the Developmental Interview (DI), the initial method for exploring and planning for your direct reports' development needs. Admittedly, developmental interviewing is a time-intensive element of leadership development, so skipping it is tempting. After its completion, however, the remaining development tasks (most of which involve regular monitoring) require much less time investment. Ultimately, the time you put into development creates the time you need to keep the effort going.

The hardest part is changing your mind-set about development so that the work becomes incorporated into your day-to-day functions, turning it into a self-reinforcing habit. We acknowledge that that is far easier said than done.

Overcoming Common Barriers

Many barriers stand between leaders and the active pursuit of development for themselves and their direct reports. The reasons range from philosophical opposition to time constraints to different organizational priorities. These justifications boil down to this: Development is not considered a critical need; thus, it loses priority to more immediate demands. Following are commonly cited reasons, along with our counter-rationale for each.

- *"We're in crisis mode. We need to put this off."* Temporary can easily turn into permanent. However, you can prevent that from happening by establishing a timeline that details the start and end dates of the delay. If you cannot commit to such a timeline, then you are likely using the "crisis" as an excuse to avoid development work altogether.
- *"My staff are self-sufficient and capable. They don't need my help with this."* Having high-performing staff does not release you from your development responsibility. During a development conversation, it is not unusual for your direct report to talk 80 percent of the time. That is to be expected; after all, this person's work and career growth are the topics. The very act of reflecting on practice can itself lead to key developmental insights.
- *"If I develop my staff, they won't stick around as long."* In reality, if a leader perceives that her superior is interested in her development, she is more likely to stick around longer rather than leave quickly. Opportunities for career growth and learning tend to engender satisfaction, trust, and loyalty.

INCORPORATING DEVELOPMENT INTO YOUR WORK

As noted earlier, the hardest part of developing others is getting to the point where it becomes routine. You can get there faster by ensuring that your approach is proactive, consistent, and efficient.

Proactive

The DI process (discussed in Chapter 5) is designed to facilitate a proactive approach because it requires those involved to specify the who, what, when, why, and how of development ahead of time. Even outside of a development agreement, you still can be proactive by

- bringing up the development subject during a scheduled or impromptu conversation with your direct report;
- adding a team process/team development discussion periodically to your regular leadership meeting agendas; and
- looking out for development-related articles, trends, and courses, and then distributing a copy or write-up to your direct reports and their staff.

Consistent

Making development part of your regular work does not mean regularly making more work for you and your direct reports. We discourage the practice of scheduling a separate meeting for the sole purpose of discussing development. Such meetings are subject to the whim of everyone's time pressures and thus become too easy to cancel. A better approach is to add development to the agenda of a standing meeting. For direct reports you do not meet with individually, plan a periodic check-in before or after a meeting that the two of you regularly attend. Consistency is critical: The more you incorporate development into your routine, the more your staff will expect it, and the more they will notice if it is falling off your radar.

Efficient

Development conversations need not take long, especially if they take place regularly. In fact, the entire cycle of bringing up the topic, getting an update, offering a suggestion, and scheduling the next progress check-in may take only ten minutes, barring any major concerns that could arise. We know of C-suite executives who hold a spontaneous "development minute" with their staff right after an implementation or a decision, to briefly reflect on lessons learned or next steps. The substance of development discussions, not the length of time, is what makes the most impact.

MONITORING DEVELOPMENT

Whether or not you use a tool such as the DI Guide (see Chapter 5), you should set up regular check-ins for monitoring and reflecting on development progress. Check-in meetings involve four stages: introduction, update, discussion, and wrap-up.

Introduction

Before the check-in, come up with a focus for the dialogue. If this is the first development meeting with your direct report, you may discuss the competency areas she needs or would like to develop. If this is a follow-up, you may ask for an update or you may go over the plans established in the DI Guide. At the end of each check-in, write a note to yourself about what was discussed or decided. That memory jog can serve as the jump-off point for the next meeting. Focus topics may include conflicts or challenges regarding a development project, contacts with key stakeholders, and accomplishments of goals. Having a focus ensures a more efficient use of your meeting time.

Update

Your direct report is in charge of giving the update about the development assignment. However, you should be an active participant, asking lead-in questions, guiding him to view alternatives, and providing advice and information when necessary. Useful questions include the following:

- How does this progress relate to your initial expectations?
  - What were the sources of the unanticipated delays? (if behind)
  - Which assumptions proved overly pessimistic? (if ahead)
- How has your understanding of (competency, department, individuals) evolved since we last met?
- At this point, what is working well or poorly? What have been the greatest challenges or surprises?

If your direct report seeks your advice on specific challenges, resist the urge to recommend specific solutions. Instead use the opportunity to develop his critical thinking skills. Help him develop approaches to a problem *similar* to the one he is facing rather than the actual one he is trying to solve. You can keep the focus on learning by first encouraging him to generate his own options for addressing the problem, adding alternatives he may not see, and then helping him select the best option. You may ask,

- What approaches do you think will work?
- What advantages and disadvantages does each method present?

Continue to help him explore the issues, expressing your insights, support, and caution along the way. If you notice blind spots, bring them up in the form of questions. For example, you may say, "It's good that you've created a detailed calendar for this new initiative. What do you think the implications of this new schedule will be on your existing initiatives and commitments?" When you think the leader is basing decisions on erroneous assumptions, be careful not to phrase your disagreement harshly. "My experience with this approach has been different. I suggest. . ." is easier to hear and thus consider than "You're definitely misjudging this method. You must. . . ."

Discussion

The discussion stage should be a mixture of constructive feedback and active questioning specifically about development. Useful questions may include the following:

- How is this assignment helping you practice and hone your competencies?
- How are you applying what you learned?
- Are you discussing your progress with your mentor (or coach)? What suggestions is your mentor giving you?
- Do you receive any other feedback? How are you using this feedback?
- Are you learning what you need to be successful? What other areas do you need to learn more about? What problems are you having a tough time with?

This exchange may reveal that some adjustments to the development plan may be needed. For example, progress may be going quicker or slower than expected, or the assignment or the mentor may prove to be a poor match. Such revisions are part of the development process, because plans need to be flexible.

Wrap-Up

End on a positive note, regardless of what transpired during the meeting. Giving a verbal pat on the back encourages not only the leader who is progressing as planned but also the direct report who is struggling to keep up. In the latter case, even if the accomplishments have been lacking, you can still say, "I appreciate your tenacity and hard work. Although we didn't reach the expected outcomes this quarter, we should look forward to a better next quarter. I am confident that you are committed to a positive outcome."

Before the meeting ends, schedule the next monitoring appointment, and jot down several ideas for discussion at the next meeting.

APPLICATION TO THE C-SUITE

Although many other leadership functions can be delegated successfully, developing your direct reports is not one of them. Lack of time is a reality for all healthcare leaders, but it should not be used as an excuse to float the feedback responsibility down to human resources, organizational development, or a hired career coach. These professionals, although capable, have a limited understanding of your direct reports' roles, styles, aspirations, and challenges. Most importantly, delegating feedback denies your leaders the benefit of your experience, perspective, and insight.

Over the years, we have seen many healthcare C-suites in which the development focus was lacking. Typical annual reviews measure the departmental or organizational achievement of balanced scorecard or dashboard metrics, but ignore the fundamental reason that these results were or were not accomplished—that is, the effectiveness or ineffectiveness of leaders and managers. Executives who regard leadership development as an investment not only start the development conversation, they also ensure that the dialogue keeps going.

REFERENCE

Economist Intelligence Unit. 2006. "The CEO's Role in Talent Management: How Top Executives from Ten Countries Are Nurturing the Leaders of Tomorrow." [Online information; retrieved 11/22/08.] www.ddiworld.com/pdf/eiu_ddi_talentmanagement_fullreport.pdf.

CHAPTER 7

Identifying and Addressing Derailment Risks

Steve, the associate vice president of medical affairs, has been working on the recruitment of a highly sought-after physician into a key service line run by Dr. Hansen. Because of some changes in the medical center's planning process, several minor aspects of the agreement had to be changed. Steve sent the changes to Allan, the senior vice president, for his signature. Allan said he needed to see Steve before signing off.

Allan: I looked carefully at the redline copy, and the contract looks fine to me. Before I sign off, I just need to confirm that you went through these changes with Dr. Hansen.

Steve: I did not. These are minor changes. They are not substantive to any of the plans that affect his service line. Also, these items are not something Dr. Hansen can negotiate about. We have to do them whether he likes it or not.

Allan: Steve, this is a much bigger issue than you seem to realize. Even if Dr. Hansen cannot affect the terms, he should have been notified. Given how some physicians react to even minor changes to an employment contract, I'll be surprised if this doesn't affect the candidate's decision to come here. If that happened, Dr. Hansen would be furious.

Steve: That's ridiculous! Why on earth would a physician make a contract decision based on something so small?

Allan: It's not the contract, Steve. It's the fact that we changed the language without telling Dr. Hansen. Put yourself in his place, and you may say to yourself, "If I can't trust the administration to be honest with me about this, what else are they going to be dishonest with me about?"

THIS VIGNETTE PORTRAYS a leader who is at risk of derailment. When a leader who was once high performing and was believed to have high potential is fired, demoted, or stalled in the same position, her career is said to have "derailed" (Lombardo and McCauley 1988). That is, she has failed to deliver the level of achievement expected for someone who had much promise.

Determining when to intervene and when to let the leader work out the problem on her own can be difficult for senior management. Stepping in is a fragile proposition: The message you communicate must be clear and strong enough that the leader understands the gravity of the situation, but it cannot be too strong that it overwhelms and drives the person to overcorrect her course.

Several factors can cause derailment, and the vignette provides an example of one of the key derailers. In this chapter, we focus on the who, what, why, and how of derailment. First, we present some reasons that leaders derail. Second, we review personal and organizational factors that serve as early warning signs (yellow flags) of current and future trouble. Third, we pose guidelines for engaging a leader in a candid discussion about derailment risks.

REASONS FOR DERAILMENT

Since the 1980s, researchers at the Center for Creative Leadership have been studying leadership derailment across various industries. Their work has identified several reasons that careers derail, including the most common one: inability to meet the performance objectives of a given role (Leslie and van Velsor 1998). On its own, failure to deliver on set objectives is the result of multiple other factors discussed in this section.

Poor Interpersonal Management

Healthcare is often described as a relationship business. As such, success in healthcare leadership positions hinges not only on well-honed interpersonal skills but also on close attention to *social capital*—a personal asset built on the quality of working relationships.

Strong interpersonal skills are part of the "entry fee" into healthcare leadership. Lack of such skills is not what derails a healthcare leader. The interpersonal problem that causes derailment is poor management of the complex dynamics inherent in group work. Conflict management is a good example. A leader who is uncomfortable with conflict may be overly accommodating. Although this approach may allow him to "keep the peace," it can prevent him from marshalling resources needed to reach performance targets.

Another dynamic is politics. In an environment of too little resources and too many priorities, give-and-take is king. That is, a leader who is always stepping over everybody else's agenda to advance her own may accomplish her goals faster and more often. However, this practice depletes this leader's social capital, which in turn harms her existing relationships and ultimately drives away the support necessary for sustainable success.

Inability to Build and Lead a Team

Effective team leadership requires highly sophisticated interpersonal skills. Assembling and managing a highly effective team requires adeptness at judging compatibility, noticing and appropriately addressing the often subtle cues of conflict, engendering a climate of open communication, and knowing when to get involved and when to grant autonomy.

Some leaders pay too little attention to whom they allow to join the team, missing out on chances to address weaknesses and blind spots when new leaders are hired. Others foster a climate in which contrarian views are discouraged or conflicts are allowed to fester unaddressed, resulting in a poor working environment and underperformance.

Difficulty Adapting to Transitions

Chapter 3 discusses the imperative for leaders to change their approach as they move from one career or life stage to the next. The derailments that occur after a transition can be attributed to a failure to recognize that old methods and perspectives will not work in the new environment. The beginning of each experience carries a substantial amount of stress; that fact alone can threaten the composure of an otherwise capable professional. For leaders who are reluctant or unable to let go of old practices and to learn new ones, the stress does not get resolved and the new position is never mastered.

YELLOW FLAGS: EARLY WARNING SIGNS OF DERAILMENT

We termed these early warning signals as "yellow flags" to indicate their propensity for turning into red flags. Although they will not necessarily lead to derailment, they pose enough of a concern to warrant careful monitoring. Sometimes, these yellow flags involve personal characteristics of the leader. Other times, they are the product of organizational realities or demands.

Personal Characteristics

Following are common individual traits that can raise a yellow flag.

Social cue illiteracy. The adage "you can't please everybody every time" applies well in healthcare leadership. Every leader has a quirk, habit, or style that charms one group but causes distress for the rest. Leaders who read social cues well know their effect on others, and many of them work on improving the qualities that others perceive negatively. Then there are the oblivious ones—senior managers who have little concept of how (well or badly) they come across. According to Gentry and colleagues (2007), leaders who do not know how others view them are at high risk for derailment because they are less likely to self-correct.

Overconfidence. Leaders need to be optimistic, but not overconfident. The most critical difference between healthy optimism and dangerous overconfidence is the capacity to hear dissenting opinions. Leaders who can acknowledge and speak convincingly to dissent are optimists, while leaders who ignore dissent are overconfident. A leader who is overconfident is reckless and risky.

Perfectionism. Many highly effective leaders are described as conscientious, meticulous, and constantly demanding excellence. The danger in these positive qualities is that they can also border on perfectionism, wherein if something is not perfect, it is worthless. Often, perfectionists alienate those around them. Perfectionist work styles that can lead to derailment include micromanagement, excessive attention to details that seem trivial, and berating staff for failing to meet standards.

Emotional volatility. All leaders experience bad days, but not all leaders lose their self-control when things do not go their way. Leaders whose emotional reactions spill into their work interactions are considered less resilient ("He is going to have a heart attack over this!"), less trustworthy ("I can't tell her about this problem. She almost fired the whole staff the last time!"), and less promotable ("If he's struggling to keep it together at this level, he's liable to come unglued at the next one!").

Organizational Characteristics

The personal characteristics discussed in the previous section coupled with deficits in management skills can create substantial organizational problems. For an in-depth discussion of these organizational yellow flags, see Finkelstein (2003). Following are five areas worth monitoring carefully.

Overly complex management structures. Although some leaders do develop highly sophisticated control systems and manage them very well, complexity can also creep into an organizational system through a series of poor decisions being layered on top of each other. A common example is a bureaucratized decision-making structure, where the levels of required permission serve more as a barrier to change or as a dodge from accountability than as an aid to decision quality. Another example is a leadership team that pushes so hard to reach consensus on every item that few decisions are made in a timely fashion, preventing them from making a significant impact.

Rapid growth. An unusually fast growth trajectory is inherently dangerous. It rapidly ushers in high volumes of new demands, which inevitably cause unanticipated problems for the service providers as well as the supporting departments. In this circumstance, the leader may not even realize that she is losing control of the work. Some warning signs include an uptick in coordination problems (e.g., important meetings are missed without explanation, essential information is not communicated to stakeholders), oversights in the physical environment (e.g., a broken clock in the waiting room that remains unfixed), and the sudden departure of one or more high-potential employees.

Excessive external involvement. Many organizations encourage their executives to be involved in professional and civic activities at the local, national, or international level. Such interests provide numerous development benefits to leaders and strengthen the organization's public image and reputation; however, over time, these external activities can draw the leader away from his organizational work. Warning signs to look for include misalignment of interests between the organization and the external group, involvement whose advantages are unclear or difficult to justify, and activities that demand substantial time but do not yield the expected benefits.

Innovation overload. Leaders who are successful organizational innovators tend to be optimists. Their confidence is essential for keeping staff's hopes up when the going gets tough. Organizations also tend to heap accolades on innovators.

However, a leader who receives early accolades for a novel idea can develop an imbalanced view, focusing increasingly on the "promise" that the initiative holds rather than maintaining an objective view of how it will work. To perpetuate the hope and the good tidings, the leader may peddle the innovation's potential and overlook concerns, even avoiding an honest discussion with his superiors. Here, the warning signs are overextended deadlines and missed goals, neither of which are adequately explained nor seem to result in appropriate levels of concern or corrections. A leader who is not fazed or at least tempered by these adverse events may not recognize when things become dire and assumptions are in need of more serious questioning.

Overemphasis on success. Healthcare executives need a powerful drive to succeed. An overemphasis on success, however, can cause problems. It results in imbalanced perspective or tunnel vision, where the leader's success is not appropriately viewed within the broader organizational context. Taken to the extreme, an overemphasis on personal success can cloud ethical judgment; this case should be considered a red, not yellow, flag that deserves immediate and forceful intervention. Signs that a leader (or the organizational culture) is too focused on pursuing success include employees who are afraid to ask questions or voice dissenting opinions and multiple comments or complaints regarding aggressive or self-serving tactics.

GUIDELINES FOR A DERAILMENT DISCUSSION

Discussing derailment is very tricky. No one, especially leaders who have repeatedly proven their knowledge and capabilities over the years, wants to hear this kind of feedback. However, it is a conversation worth having, as it can make the difference between good leadership and exceptional leadership, both for yourself and your struggling direct report. Following are guidelines for conducting such a discussion.

First, however, a note about preparation. You should enter this conversation as well equipped with information and strategies as possible. After all, a derailment discussion is not a routine check-in. Even the approach you take in scheduling this appointment is critical. If the problem is minor, it may be addressed during the next development meeting. If the concern is substantial, it should be dealt with as soon as possible; preempt an existing appointment if necessary. Scheduling a special meeting accomplishes two goals: (1) it allows a timely, focused response to the situation, and (2) it draws attention to the significance of the problem. The end of the workday or workweek is ideal for this discussion because it gives the leader time to reflect afterward, outside the organization's walls.

Clarify the Concern Ahead of Time

The struggling leader is likely not aware of his own predicament, so before the meeting you should lay out the specifics, which will ensure you are both on the same page:

- Review the leader's job expectations and responsibilities.
- Identify the critical incident(s) (e.g., situation, decision, action, or inaction).
- Describe the ideal approach to the scenario, then compare it to the method the leader actually used.
- Note the immediate outcomes and the long-term implications of the leader's approach.
- Articulate the consequences and risks to the leader's long-term performance.
- Recommend a pathway to improvement, with a timeline.

Follow a Structure

Prevent any risk of interruption by nonemergency phone calls, e-mails, tasks, or visits. Close the door, and, if necessary, turn off your mobile communication devices.

At the start, set a tone of positive reflection. Together, you may talk about the experiences and development the leader has experienced during his tenure, then gradually move on to his future career plans, keeping the mood congenial but focused. The point of this exercise is to put the leader at ease for the oncoming constructive feedback and to get him to adopt a long-term perspective for its implications.

The next step is to gently, but firmly, lay your concerns on the table. Frame this discussion in terms of how the problem is interfering with his and the organization's success. During the conversation, pause to solicit feedback, clarification, or contribution from the leader. Do not turn the session into an interrogation, however. Listen intently to his input, and reflect on it afterward. Model the behavior you would like to see if you were in his shoes.

No matter how much groundwork you have laid, you should expect a rough or unsteady session. The leader may react defensively, expressing his frustrations and arguing his side of the story.

Allow him to air out his thoughts, and express understanding for the challenges he faces. If he continues to be aggressive and does not accept the feedback, then simply stop the conversation, saying: "It's best that we continue this discussion at another time. Please give some thought to this situation and how we can improve it. More than anything, we both can't afford to find ourselves several months in the future wondering what we could have done today to fix this problem."

Providing the discussion goes as planned, move on to discuss improvement plans and set a follow-up appointment. End the session by expressing your appreciation for the leader's time, openness to feedback, and willingness to take positive steps toward improvement.

APPLICATION TO THE C-SUITE

Derailment is particularly acute in the C-suite. At this level, feedback on interpersonal practices and leadership competencies is often sparse or absent. Without this kind of feedback, senior leaders lose perspective and develop harmful tendencies such as overconfidence, tunnel vision, and even emotional volatility.

Senior executives who are new to an organization also face a higher risk of derailment. These leaders are placed under immense pressure to establish legitimacy quickly. Meeting this expectation can create problems, which are in turn masked until the leader begins to spiral out of control. For these executives, the best treatment is prevention. First, they should be given proper supervision for the first several months on the job. Second, if a search consultant was involved in the recruitment, that consultant should act as a conduit between the organization and the newly hired leader, clarifying expectations and responsibilities. Third, an astute chief human resources officer should help ease the leader into her new role by routinely checking in. Finally, during the first year, the executive should be encouraged to engage other senior leaders in her decision-making processes. By offering guidance and support to the new leader, you are helping her to be fully competent, knowledgeable, and in charge amid any pressure situations.

The best approach to heading off derailment is to include an interpersonal section in executive performance reviews. This section can be informed by 360-degree evaluations or other such assessments facilitated by a neutral outsider. An external coach, which many organizations offer to their senior management team, can ensure that the leader hears and uses interpersonal feedback from peers and direct reports.

REFERENCES

Finkelstein, S. 2003. *Why Smart Executives Fail*. New York: Portfolio.

Gentry, W. A., K. M. Hannum, B. Z. Ekelund, and A. de Jong. 2007. "A Study of the Discrepancy Between Self- and Observer-Ratings on Managerial Derailment Characteristics of European Managers." *European Journal of Work and Organizational Psychology* 16 (3): 295–325.

Leslie, J. B., and F. van Velsor. 1998. *A Look at Derailment Today: North America and Europe*. Greensboro, NC: Center for Creative Leadership.

Lombardo, M. M., and C. D. McCauley. 1988. *The Dynamics of Management Derailment*. Greensboro, NC: Center for Creative Leadership.

CHAPTER 8

Managing Transitions

Marianna just accepted an offer for a CEO position in another state. In the last ten years, she worked under Ruth, the system's CEO, who provided much advocacy and support. Under Ruth, Marianna fully developed as a leader, receiving two promotions, exposure to the board, and opportunities to negotiate several physician contracts and joint ventures.

When Marianna approached Ruth about her resignation, Ruth seemed uncomfortable, muttering a half-hearted congratulations, avoiding eye contact, and offering no real support or encouragement. Marianna came prepared to discuss a transition plan, but she decided to postpone this discussion given Ruth's reaction. Disappointed, Marianna called Bill, her search consultant, to seek advice on how to manage her departure and salvage her relationship with Ruth.

Bill: These situations are rarely easy. You have described Ruth to me as valuing loyalty above all else. In hindsight, she would have likely preferred that you spoke to her before you made a decision—to ask for her blessing, so to speak, or at least to allow her to weigh in.

Marianna: I wanted to, but I was afraid she would pressure me to stay. I would not have been able to make a clear-minded decision had I approached her first.

Bill: I can understand that. Here's a suggestion: Wait a couple of days for this news to sink in, and then schedule another meeting with Ruth. Bring a small gift, a token of your appreciation. Be honest about how you made your decision, and apologize that your announcement caught her off guard. Emphasize how grateful you are for all her help throughout the years. Most importantly, express your wish that she can come to accept your decision as you would welcome her continued guidance for your new challenge. How does that sound?

Marianna: I like it, and I think Ruth will, too. I will let you know how our next meeting goes. Thanks.

THIS VIGNETTE ILLUSTRATES an organizational truism: Poorly executed leadership transitions can damage even the most stable relationships. Transitions are a regular part of work life, and they are an inevitable product of career growth and development. Managing them effectively is a hallmark of excellent leadership and demonstrates the executive's balance and maturity under pressure.

This chapter provides a broad treatment of transitions, both outgoing and incoming. First, we review the reasons that leaders pursue other opportunities. Second, we offer strategies to ease the transition, not only of your direct reports but also your own. Third, we present practices for appropriately initiating new hires and promotions, approaches that you may also apply to your own moves.

REASONS FOR DEPARTURE

From the perspective of the executive search field, leaders are interested in position moves if the new position meets a combination of three criteria: better compensation, better opportunity, and better location.

A departing leader may be attracted by higher compensation. An organization may place more value on the same position the leader holds, or the position may involve different or greater responsibilities. In either case, if the main motivation is money, the leader may be driven either by the need for increased resources or an interest in a higher standard of living.

Better opportunity is typically represented by a position that enables the leader to gain different experiences or to expand responsibilities. Leaders also seek new opportunities if they believe their current role is not a good fit for their abilities. Sometimes, a leader will take another position simply for the chance to face a different set of challenges or to work in a different setting.

Better location is the most immutable of these three reasons, because the underlying factors here are typically personal. Relocation is most frequently motivated by a desire to be closer to family or relatives (e.g., aging parents, recently born grandchildren).

GRACEFUL GOOD-BYES

Several strategies can help a smooth transition for the departing leader and the organization.

Contain Your Initial Reaction

An unexpected announcement of a departure can stir feelings of betrayal and defensiveness, particularly if the leader has never even mentioned looking at other opportunities. This news is especially difficult to accept when it comes from a high-potential leader, from someone in a mission-critical or difficult-to-fill post, or during an already stressful time. Dread or panic may set in, as you ask yourself, "How on earth can I refill this role?"

All such reactions are natural. However, be cautious about how you express them because your initial response can make the difference between a smooth and a contentious transition.

Check your reaction by reminding yourself of the following realities.

- *All positions are finite.* No one person can fill a role forever. That person will eventually leave through his own or another's decision. Indeed, stronger leaders and better development climates—both good things—will also yield more rapid position changes. The most talented leaders tend to progress up the career ladder faster, so brace yourself for that eventuality.

- *A transition is always a mixed blessing.* Every leader, no matter how talented, has development needs and blind spots, in addition to strengths. Although losing a good leader inevitably disrupts your momentum, it also presents the opportunity for a fresh perspective and new direction. For any departing leader, it is possible to honestly express both sadness and optimism.

Create a Transition Plan

The time between a leader's resignation and departure should be viewed as a precious resource, not to be squandered by "writing off" the leader. Working up a plan for using this resource can yield maximum benefits for the organization and the affected staff.

Prioritize ongoing projects. Ask the leader to make a list of all her current projects. Discuss this list with her, asking relevant questions (requirements, goals, timelines, key players) about each item. Rank order the list according to importance and the need for the leader to be involved. Negotiate with her a reasonable set of projects to complete before her last day. Sometimes, leaders in this situation feel guilty about leaving and thus overcommit to finishing current projects. Help her keep her commitments realistic. Finally, ask her to summarize this discussion in writing so that you can both refer to it later.

Plan for post-transition communications. Departing leaders almost always take with them critical but undocumented knowledge and information. Therefore, explicitly ask the leader for permission to contact him if necessary. Also, request that he grant you a follow-up call when his replacement is named so that he may share insights from his experiences in the role.

This request is more likely to receive a "yes" if you first offer to help him during the pivotal early months on his new role. If the leader hesitates about continuing a dialogue or guiding your new hire, then inquire about his concerns or barriers and suggest some parameters that will address them. For example, if he is concerned about work-hours contact, offer to only call before or after regular working hours; if the new employer is a competitor, agree to set some topics as out of bounds.

Publicly Recognize the Transition

Regardless of the circumstance of the departure, the message communicated to the staff should convey that (1) the leader's talents and contributions are greatly appreciated and will be missed and that (2) a solid plan is in place that will ensure continuity of work during and after the transition period. Good-bye events, such as a lunch or an evening reception, can be an effective way not only to celebrate the leader but also to recognize your other staff's hard work and dedication. If feasible, invite managers, support staff, and clinicians throughout the organization with whom the leader worked closely during her tenure.

MANAGING YOUR OWN EXIT

The approaches presented thus far also apply to your own departure. As a senior executive, however, your career move will involve additional considerations, not the least of which is whether or not to inform your superior of your interest in other opportunities. See Figure 8.1 for guidelines about this sensitive issue.

Figure 8.1 Decision-Making Guidelines for a Transition: To Tell or Not to Tell

Open dialogue is essential for effective development. When it comes to leadership transitions, however, honesty is not always the best policy. Consider the following before you discuss an interest in moving on:

- *How did my superior react to similar announcements and transitions?* Some chief executives value loyalty and devotion above all else. They talk viciously about people who left their posts, sometimes for years afterward. If this describes your superior, then stating your intention to leave is a bad idea, as you may get the same treatment even before you go.
- *What are my prospects for promotion if I stay?* If you have had ongoing conversations with your boss about your career goals and have come to the conclusion that moving up the organizational hierarchy is not a possibility, then your boss may be more amenable to and supportive of your decision to seek other opportunities.
- *How serious am I about moving on?* The more seriously you are taking your job search, the more reason you have to discuss it with your superior. However, if interviewing for jobs is merely a casual habit that produces no results, then telling your boss will only make you seem less dedicated to your current role or uncertain about your career.
- *How easy/difficult will it be to replace me?* A superior will be rightly concerned about the onus of replacing you and the demands that will entail. If you have prepared a direct report well to step up to your role, then the news of your potential departure should seem less threatening.

Once you have made a decision to leave, we recommend the following next steps.

Give Ample Notice

The pressure to start your new role right away may be enormous. However, you should consider it your professional duty to leave behind a firm foundation for the next executive and the remaining staff. Also, keep in mind that the leaders of your new organization should allow you to take a reasonable amount of time to transition, as they would likely prefer the same treatment from their own departing leaders.

Carefully Plan the Announcement

Your transition will entail a substantial change, especially because of the relationships you have forged with your direct reports. Your staff's reaction to the news may vary, from accepting to resentful. Some may even feel abandoned.

After informing your superior, you should schedule a meeting with each of your direct reports. The next two conversations you should have are (1) with your successor (if already selected) or the person who will fill your role in the interim and (2) with other members of the senior management team. These meetings should occur quickly because word about your departure may spread rapidly after your initial announcements.

Prepare for these departure discussions, especially the one with your staff. Use this opportunity to extend your gratitude for their support, to express your faith in their continued career growth and development, and to recognize their professional accomplishments.

Touch Base "Backwards"

Despite the hectic schedule of your new role, make time to check in, even if only briefly, with your former direct reports and associates. For example, three to four weeks after your departure, call your previous boss with an offer to give advice or insight to your replacement. Also, update your address, phone, and e-mail lists so that you may continue to send greeting cards or notes to friends from your prior organization. In whatever form of contact you choose, do not gloat about better conditions in your new position, regardless of the truth. Balance upsides with downsides in any descriptions you provide. The point here is to maintain the goodwill and working relationships you developed over many years.

HELPFUL HELLOS

The first 90 days of a leadership role are often intense. This is the period in which you must form new relationships, develop and internalize a mental model of the organization, and clarify short- and long-term objectives.

During this time, new leaders are typically given more benefit than doubt, a resource that may be squandered or applied strategically. We all recognize that learning the formal and informal rules of the organization takes some time, and slip-ups are generally forgiven. In any case, successful leaders do not get distracted or caught up in the excitement of the transition and are not lulled into a false sense of confidence in their early days. Instead, they plan their starts appropriately to get the maximum benefit from the grace period.

Following are strategies for navigating your or your leader's first 90 days. For more in-depth discussions of these transitional periods, see Watkins (2003) and Ciampa and Watkins (1999).

Set Clear End and Start Dates

End and start dates are easier to establish if the transition involves a move to a different organization. However, they are still important to set even if the transition is internal—that is, a promotion within the organization or department.

Draw attention to an internal transition by setting and communicating specific transition dates and transition events. For example, on the last day of the old role you could take the promoted leader to a favorite restaurant to celebrate, and use the time to reflect on the old role and plan for the new one. On the transition day, set aside time to discuss with the leader her new responsibilities and the plans for delegating existing assignments to her replacement.

Assess the Role

If the new leader was an external recruit, the interview and selection processes should have painted a broad picture of the role's expectations. As the superior, your job is to help the new leader fill in the details. That is, the new leader has to thoroughly evaluate the position, gathering as much data and information as possible, to answer the question, What needs to be done here? This analysis, in turn, will inform the new leader's 90-day plan and will help steer longer-term plans. This process also applies to your own transition.

Size Up Your Direct Reports

The new leader should determine the performance levels and abilities of his immediate staff. Typically a leader will find that some employees outperform the others, while some need guidance and improvement in specific areas. Another frequent discovery is that direct reports' capabilities are misaligned with their roles, requiring more immediate intervention.

Encourage the leader to meet with each of his staff members to get a sense of personalities, abilities, and career goals. He may want to hold off on conducting a developmental interview (see Chapter 5) until he has a clearer sense of whom he will want to keep, but some of the questions in the Developmental Interview Guide (see Appendix A) may help in getting to know the staff. Particularly useful are questions about their current position, length of service, and career trajectory.

In addition, assist the leader in identifying individuals in each department with whom he will regularly interface, either as strategic partners or as sources of support. On his own, he may want to ask colleagues whom they consider the "go-to" people, then note these names.

Identify Initial Goals

After a diagnosis of the environment, the job, and the direct reports, the new leader should prioritize her first projects:

- *"Easy wins."* These are issues that cause widespread aggravation but are relatively straightforward to resolve. For example, some unit processes may have outlived their effectiveness and have become a source of extra work and thus annoyance. Streamlining such processes will earn the new leader credibility among staff and set her momentum as a change agent.
- *Larger, higher-visibility changes.* Early goals should also include visible headway on the core expectations of the role. What are the areas of underperformance that she can influence the most? What are the main barriers to progress, and how can she overcome them?

Build Mission-Critical Relationships

The new leader should seek out opportunities to work with, and ideally help out, the key people she will later rely on for her future plans. This step is critical for a leader who just entered the organization, but it is equally important for a promoted leader because the nature of his interpersonal exchanges will likely need to evolve.

Write a 90-Day Report

Required or not, writing a 90-day report is a beneficial exercise. It serves at least two purposes. First, it forces the leader to articulate her initial diagnoses and future plans. Second, it can be used to assess the alignment between the leader's perspectives and those of her superior. The report should include (1) an assessment of the current situation, which is informed by data the leader has gathered; (2) the direction she plans to take forward; and (3) a prioritized list of next steps.

As the superior, you should discuss parts of the plan about which you and the leader do not see eye-to-eye. This discussion can help address blind spots in the new leader's understanding of the organization, but be aware that, during this talk, your new leader may see aspects of the organization to which you have become blind. A revision or a compromise may be necessary to bridge your differences.

APPLICATION TO THE C-SUITE

Surveys suggest that most healthcare CEOs do not believe their organizations effectively communicate about leadership transitions (e.g., Garman and Tyler 2007). This finding is disturbing because people often regard the stability of the senior management team as an indicator of the overall organization's stability. For this reason, transitions within the C-suite must be cautiously managed, with a focus on clear communication.

Following are key strategies related to managing and communicating a transition.

- *Keep the process transparent.* All key stakeholders (e.g., staff, physicians, board) should be informed about the succession or transition process. Afterward, a general, not detailed, update should be regularly provided and available as part of your regular organizational communication channels (e.g., intranet, management briefings).
- *Keep the communications consistent.* Take steps to ensure that board members and other key stakeholders convey a uniform message. This helps to underscore that the process being followed is thoughtful and methodical.
- *Keep employees informed.* Employees should always hear about transitions from organizational leaders rather than from the media. Build internal communications into all critical stages of dissemination to ensure that employees hear from you first.
- *Capitalize on media attention.* Encourage your public relations team to proactively inform the media so that the team has more control over the message. The team may emphasize the positive evolution of leadership, or it may steer the reporters toward featuring innovations as a representation of positive strides the organization has taken in serving its community.

REFERENCES

Ciampa, D., and M. Watkins. 1999. *Right from the Start: Taking Charge in a New Leadership Role.* Boston: Harvard Business School Press.

Garman, A. N., and J. L. Tyler. 2007. "Succession Planning Practices and Outcomes in U.S. Hospital Systems: Final Report." [Online information; retrieved 9/1/08.] www.ache.org/pubs/research/succession_planning.pdf.

Watkins, M. 2003. *The First 90 Days: Critical Success Strategies for New Leaders at All Levels.* Boston: Harvard Business School Press.

CHAPTER 9

Fostering an Organizational Approach to Leadership Development

Kevin is one of three assistant vice presidents in the support services department. His boss, Angelo, recently announced that he is leaving to fill a post in another organization. Immediately after hearing this news, Kevin requested a meeting with Maureen, the chief administrative officer, to discuss the possibility of moving into Angelo's position.

The meeting between Kevin and Maureen began cordially, with Maureen complimenting Kevin on the outstanding work he has delivered in his two-year tenure. However, the conversation then took an unexpected turn.

Kevin: I asked Angelo outright if I was next in line for his job. He said the decision wasn't his to make, but he offered to walk me through the skills I need to strengthen or develop if I wanted to move into the role.

Maureen: That's a good start. What did he propose?

Kevin: We didn't get that far. I wasn't looking for a coaching session. I wanted him to cut to the chase.

Maureen: He is right that he is not the decision maker, but he does have input into the replacement process. Because he knows his direct reports much better than I do, I asked him to summarize each of the assistant vice presidents' strengths and limitations using the competencies for that position. The input Angelo provided then helps our decision making.

Kevin: "Our" decision making? I don't understand. Isn't all this going to be your call at the end of the day?

Maureen: An internal committee handles these transitions. I'm on the committee, and so are several other senior leaders.

Kevin: I mean no disrespect, but this group seems just another way to diffuse responsibility for hard decisions. You don't strike me as someone who backs away from making tough calls!

Maureen: This committee is not about diffusing responsibility. It allows us to broaden our succession approach by collecting objective input and assessing our available options. Ultimately, the decisions we make through this process will best serve the organization's long-term interests.

Kevin: Again, let's cut to the chase here.

Maureen: We will review your profile, along with those of the other two assistant vice presidents and even qualified candidates who are not Angelo's direct reports.

Kevin: Well, that hardly seems fair! I busted my tail in this position, but now I could lose my break to someone who has not even set foot into this department. This system sounds like a bunch of political BS!

Maureen: We need to end this conversation, Kevin. I have given you the information you have come to discuss. But in defense of this process, I must say that it is more fair than the political posturing this organization has practiced for many years. Regardless of your personal views, this system focuses on demonstrated outcomes and capabilities, not merely on relationships or length of service. It does not operate under the blind assumption that a leadership role could be handed to whoever is around to fill it. The committee works hard to assess the required competencies for each role. For a better understanding of those competencies, I will refer you back to Angelo's offer of assistance.

Kevin: Maureen, I apologize for the tone of my reaction. I need some time to think this through.

Maureen: I can appreciate that you take your career seriously,

Kevin. Angelo is going to be here for four more weeks. I suggest you have that development discussion with him while you still can.

THIS VIGNETTE DESCRIBES a change from the way leadership development has been approached historically in healthcare organizations. In the past, promotions relied heavily on individual accomplishments, relationships, or seniority, rather than on objective competency-based measures.

This chapter explores the ideas introduced in the vignette, describing a leadership development process that supports and forwards organizational, not just individual, goals. We make the case that an organizational approach to development does not overshadow the need for superiors to develop their direct reports. Rather, it complements individual-development efforts. Also, we enumerate the practices that can extend the reach of leadership development.

LEADERSHIP, NOT LEADER, DEVELOPMENT

Raising the rank of leadership development on the organization's priority list is a struggle for many executives. In a survey of healthcare leaders, more than two-thirds of respondents believed that their organization's approach to preparing leaders for promotions was not effective. However, fewer than 1 percent of study participants said that they thought succession planning process was not useful (Garman and Tyler 2006). To help senior management advance leadership development within their organizations, a clarification is in order.

Leader development is distinct from *leadership* development (see Table 9.1). The former emphasizes the individual, while the

Table 9.1 Leader Development and Leadership Development: Similarities and Differences

Dimension	Leader Development	Leadership Development
Goals	• Improving an individual leader's effectiveness • Keeping a high-potential leader engaged and developing • Enhancing a leader's readiness for promotion	• Improving organizational effectiveness • Attracting talented leaders to the organization • Keeping high-potential leaders engaged and developing • Developing and communicating career paths • Enhancing the "bench strength" of next-generation leaders
Focus	• The individual leader	• Leaders as a collective network
Oversight and Decision Making	• Individual leader; the leader in collaboration with superior	• Team-based; steering committee or other oversight group in addition to development participants

Table 9.1 continued

Formal Strategies	• Individual attendance at off-site programs (e.g., workshops, seminars, and conferences) • Individual attendance at organization-sponsored internal workshops • Enrollment in courses and degree programs • Team attendance at off-site programs (e.g., workshops, seminars, and conferences) • Group/team attendance at on-site customized workshops • Internal leadership development programs
Informal or On-the-Job Strategies	• Individual development plan • Job/project assignment • Individual feedback • Executive coaching • Peer evaluation • Group process consultation • Action-learning assignment • 360-degree feedback • Developmental Assessment Center
Basis for Evaluation	• Improvements in individual performance • Support for organizational goals

latter focuses on the group. Effective leadership development binds leader development activities into an integrated whole and is directly linked to organization-level goals.

Broadening the Definition of Successful Leadership

In healthcare, success is often defined at the individual level, which makes sense for measuring the leader's performance. For example, we may define Mary's success in terms of whether her service line reached its volume targets, or we may gauge Joe's achievements by whether or not he came in at or under budget for his support department. This individual definition only refers to the "what," not the "how."

In contrast, a broad definition involves the "how" or the process followed to pursue success. Are we going to emphasize collaboration or competition? Should we focus on making decisions quickly, or on pursuing consensus? Which should take precedence: critical debate or keeping the peace?

The competency models discussed in Chapter 1 can function as a starting point for redefining successful leadership. An even more useful tool is a competency model that has been customized to reflect the perspectives of your organization's leadership. An organization-specific model provides a solid foundation for other systemwide leadership development activities, which are aligned with senior leadership's mind-set.

APPROACHES TO LEADERSHIP DEVELOPMENT

Following are competency-based practices that can expand development beyond individual leaders.

Multisource Feedback

Multisource feedback (or 360-degree feedback) involves collecting from various sources (e.g., superiors, peers, direct reports, clients) performance-related information about a particular leader. This feedback is usually obtained through an electronic survey. Respondent input is then aggregated into a summary report that disguises the sources, allowing participant feedback to remain anonymous.

For example, an organization's competency model may include "earning loyalty and trust." Respondents may be asked to rate the leader on his effectiveness in this competency, with "10" indicating a top mark and "1" signaling a serious concern. Respondents may also be given an opportunity to elaborate on their ranking by describing specific past events or suggestions for improvement; for example, "You have lost trust in the past by making decisions that you failed to communicate to people who were affected. The laboratory space project comes immediately to mind."

Although the main focus of multisource feedback is the individual leader, the technique can be even more powerful when applied to leadership development. If a leadership team participates in multisource feedback together, then team-level results can be calculated, and systemic strengths and weaknesses can be identified and addressed. For example, if "earning loyalty and trust" is, on average, the lowest-rated competency for all leaders who have received a 360-degree feedback, then organizational practices associated with corporate communications, transparency, and equity should be examined. (Appendix F of Dye and Garman [2006] provides a guide for implementing 360-degree feedback.)

Group Process Consultation

Committee work is a common example of an activity that distinguishes leadership development from leader development. For many leadership teams, the time pressure on agendas and decision making is relentless. In this climate, finding the time to collectively reflect on how decisions are made, how groups are structured, or how agendas are set up can seem futile. This is true even when everyone in the group agrees that the group's approach to the work is coming up short. The bottom line remains: We have to finish the budget, or prepare for the Joint Commission visit, and so on.

Group process consultation is a viable approach in such an environment. In this process, a facilitator—someone who is not a member of the group—attends a series of team meetings to observe the approaches used. Typically, the facilitator first surveys the team, asking each member to identify what works well and to recommend improvements to what does not work. The findings are then fed back to the group, and the facilitator encourages and helps the team to change one or more areas. Over the next several meetings, the facilitator watches for improvements in the problem areas identified, bringing them to the group's attention as needed. For example, if the committee is working on improving accountability, the consultant may point out decisions in which the responsible parties or timelines have not been identified. Although the consultant may comment on an individual's actions or inactions, the focus is on the performance of the group as a whole.

Process consultation can offer fresh perspectives on habits that have become ingrained over the years. Working with a skilled facilitator can quickly yield substantial benefits. Our experience has shown that the lessons learned with this method are applicable beyond the group; they can be carried back to members' own departments and meetings.

Reflective Learning Forum

The idea behind a *reflective learning forum* is to discuss leadership activities and knowledge for the purpose of peer learning. Forums can be structured in a number of ways. One practice is *management grand rounds,* a periodic meeting, similar to clinical grand rounds, in which leaders convene to address an organizational issue or challenge. Another example is a *learning forum,* a peer-led discussion of a topic relevant to the organization. Typically, these forums meet not less than once a quarter but not more than once a month. Members rotate responsibility for the meeting content, which may involve a discussion of a book or an article related to the issue at hand and a guest speaker who can provide insights about the topic of the meeting. Learning forums are also useful for bringing together subgroups of leaders—for example, early careerists; women or minority groups; high-potential leaders; or leaders with specific interests, such as the environment or community outreach.

Talent Review

Talent review is a periodic (often annual) meeting to examine the performance of the leadership teams in the organization. Here, individual and collective leadership needs or gaps are identified. This review typically involves several executives, including the superior of the leadership group, a representative from the human resources department (usually the chief human resources officer), and/or an outside consultant. The Nine-Box Technique discussed in Chapter 1 is often used to frame the talent review process.

If talent review is adopted throughout the organization, the process can become a tool for aligning leadership development with organizational goals. In particular, talent reviews can help identify high-potential leaders in other parts of the organization who may be excellent candidates for senior roles in other areas. The talent review can illuminate potential organization-wide development paths that would otherwise remain invisible.

TOWARD LEADERSHIP DEVELOPMENT

How an organization graduates from an informal, decentralized leader development process to a systematic, centralized leader*ship* approach is never an accident. This evolution is deliberate, usually involving the phases discussed in this section.

The Case for Change

As with all other initiatives, leadership development is sparked by a "burning platform," a compelling case for change. Following are several common catalysts for this change.

Succession crisis. In this instance, a CEO or other key leader unexpectedly leaves, becomes suddenly ill, or passes away, causing the remaining C-suite leaders and the board to scramble for a replacement. This crisis opens a window of opportunity for discussing the implementation of a more systematic approach to succession planning. (For a concise, board-appropriate article summarizing the barriers to executive-level succession planning, see Figure 9.1 at the end of this chapter.)

Looming mass retirement. An analysis of the demographic composition of employees often reveals that expected retirement dates are not evenly distributed. That is, a substantial number of leaders will potentially retire at about the same time. Organizations with long-tenure leaders may also be at risk for cohort turnover, whereby one leader's retirement highly influences her peers' decisions ("Rebecca's retiring, so it must be time for me to retire as well").

Diversity imperative. An analysis of the workforce demographics may lead to a realization that the composition of the current leadership team does not reflect that of the service population, and it never will unless actions are taken. This finding is a compelling case to increase attention to diversity in hiring and to prepare diverse leaders at lower levels for positions of greater responsibility.

Turnover of high-potentials. The loss of several high-potential leaders can cause senior leaders to recognize that their organization is underperforming in attracting, promoting, or retaining talent. Exit interviews may reveal a pattern of frustration with advancement and development. In these cases, a greater focus on leadership development may emphasize retention as much as performance improvement.

The Culture Shift

Culture shifts are most successfully introduced by a new board member or an incoming executive who has experience in other organizations that strongly emphasized leadership development. This leader then takes on the enormous task of educating his peers and being the champion for change.

A cultural shift necessitates more than merely communicating and selling the new approach. It also entails planning, development, implementation, and monitoring, all of which take several years. For example, if an organization adopts a leadership core competency model in 2008, it may not use that model to support voluntary leadership development activities until 2009. Implementing a new hiring and talent review processes may not occur until 2010.

Goal Alignment

For leadership development to get and stay off the ground, its outcomes must be measurable. Many organizations accomplish this by aligning the program goals with one or more corporate goals; management retention and employee satisfaction/engagement are two common examples. Other metrics include adequacy of succession plans (e.g., the number of key leadership positions for which at least one internal candidate is ready now to step into if needed) and percentage of management positions filled by internal promotions.

APPLICATION TO THE C-SUITE

C-suite executives have a compelling opportunity, and responsibility, to foster an organizational leadership development approach, extending their reach beyond their own direct reports. Leadership development programs are almost always most effective when originated by the C-suite team, as these leaders are the role models for the rest of the organization. Half-hearted attempts by senior management result in no cultural transformation and little implementation anywhere else.

By collaboratively discussing development needs and promotion opportunities across the system and by assessing their own strengths and weaknesses, senior leaders communicate their commitment to the program. Consequently, the pathways to organization-wide leadership development are cleared and become easier to follow. Board support and involvement are also important. If leadership development and succession planning are not part of the board's agenda, include them in the board's ongoing education. See Figure 9.1 for insight into the board's role in succession planning.

REFERENCES

Dye, C. F., and A. N. Garman. 2006. *Exceptional Leadership: 16 Critical Competencies for Healthcare Executives.* Chicago: Health Administration Press.

Garman, A. N. 2005. "Why Succession Planning May Not Be on Your Board's Agenda, But Should Be." *Boardroom Press.* [Online information; retrieved 11/1/08.] www.governanceinstitute.com/LinkClick.aspx?fileticket=eLoRr2ANMH8%3d& tabid=185&forcedownload=true.

Garman, A. N., and J. L. Tyler. 2006. *Succession Planning Practices and Outcomes in U.S. Hospital Systems: Final Report.* [Online information; retrieved 6/1/08.] www.ache.org/pubs/research/succession_planning.pdf.

Figure 9.1 Why Succession Planning May Not Be on Your Board's Agenda—But Should Be

Does your board have a succession plan in place for the incumbent CEO? If not, you have lots of company, but it's not necessarily good company.

In November 2004, the American College of Healthcare Executives (ACHE) released results of a national study of CEO succession planning in freestanding hospitals (see the full report at www.ache.org/pubs/research/ SuccessionRpt04.pdf). With 722 hospitals participating, the study may be the most comprehensive look at national succession planning practices ever published. The big-picture finding: Only 15 percent of respondents said they have a successor identified for the incumbent CEO.

Why have so few boards implemented succession plans? According to the survey, it was not for lack of interest (only 1 percent of respondents without succession plans said they thought the process wasn't useful). The four most frequently cited barriers were (1) the CEO was too new, (2) there was lack of internal candidates to prepare, (3) it was not a high enough priority, and (4) it was not a part of the organization's culture.

Barrier 1: The CEO Was Too New
If a CEO is relatively new to the role, succession planning could seem premature at best; at worst, board members may worry that forcing the issue may be interpreted by the CEO as a lack of confidence in his/her abilities. Although the concern may be valid, it should be weighed carefully against the risks of continuing without a plan. To see why, consider how long it takes to fully prepare a successor to assume the CEO role. Prevailing expert opinions as well as the results of this recent study suggest it can take

Figure 9.1 continued

as long as four to five years. When you consider that the average CEO tenure is not much longer than this preparation time, it becomes clear that succession planning works best as a continuous process.

Barrier 2: Lack of Internal Candidates to Prepare
The board and CEO may believe that no one in the senior management team has the capacity to eventually assume the CEO role. About one in four of the respondents in the ACHE survey indicated this was a barrier in their own institutions. In these cases, the option that seemed best was to wait until a new CEO was needed and then fill the position via external search.

However, this strategy is not without serious risk for several reasons. First, the ACHE study revealed a substantial "cohort effect" in CEOs—many will be retiring at the same time. As a result, shuffling the remaining candidates will not cover the vacancies; many replacements will need to be groomed from the management layers below.

But even if your hospital is successful in attracting outside talent, there are other challenges an outsider would face. Reflect for a moment on the amount of social and political capital your current CEO has developed over the course of her tenure. Consider how long it took to develop that capital and the amount of time and energy it would take a newcomer (perhaps even someone from outside your community) to cultivate those relationships.

Many CEOs identified by external search struggle in their new roles, even if they were performing effectively in their prior organizations. Other things being roughly equal, an internal candidate who knows the organization well (and, more important, is trusted by key stakeholders) will have an easier time focusing his energy on the work to be done and be spared the need to build relationships and navigate political waters anew.

Barrier 3: Not a High Enough Priority
The most frequent barrier in this study, cited by almost half the respondents, was that succession planning just was not a high enough priority. Given the near-term pressures constantly facing boards, it may be difficult

Figure 9.1 continued

to make time on the agenda for a regular succession planning process, particularly when the CEO is doing well and is nowhere near retirement age.

But consider what would cause succession planning to come to the board's attention. In the best of all possible circumstances, it would involve a well-performing CEO preparing for his/her retirement, working with the board to identify a successor, and then grooming that successor to assume the role at a predetermined date at least four years down the road. However, a lot can go wrong on the way to that scenario, much of it outside of the board and the CEO's control: illness, untimely demise, unexpected turnover, performance declines, and changing strategic needs, to name a few. An ongoing succession planning process is as much about the unanticipated as it is the anticipated needs.

Barrier 4: Not a Part of the Organization's Culture
More than one in five respondents indicated that succession planning was not a part of the culture of their organizations. In other words, it was not routine practice, not viewed as essential to success. To us, this suggests that succession planning is not a part of the roles for governance. Considering all of the reasons stated above, it needs to be. Not only is succession planning for the incumbent CEO and his/her actual successor vital to the continuous governance process, it demonstrates sound planning practices.

Source: Andrew N. Garman, PsyD, MS, "Why Succession Planning May Not Be on Your Board's Agenda—But Should Be," *BoardRoom Press*, Volume 16, No. 2, April 2005, The Governance Institute. Used with permission.

PART III

CHAPTER 10

Supporting the Development of Diverse Leaders

Mary, the chief human resources officer for Alpha Health System, just finished her annual update on the organization's talent management program. Her audience consisted of Bob, the system CEO; Susan, the chair of the board's human resources committee and a former human resources officer for a *Fortune* 500 firm; and Edward, the chair of the board. Over the past two years, the system's talent management program has evolved to incorporate succession and transition planning and targeted diversity hiring. Mary articulated future plans to shift attention back to internal training resources and career pathing. She also gave an in-depth review of the diversity hiring plan, mentioning that the current candidate pools are measurably diverse and that diversity hiring has gone up. Afterward, she welcomed questions and comments.

Susan: Thank you for an informative presentation! Is there a specific reason that you focused only on hiring rather than on leadership team composition and turnover? I know that your complete report includes these numbers, but what is your opinion on the fact that turnover among diverse leaders is high and that the movement of diverse candidates into leadership positions is going very slowly at best?

Bob: I'd like to respond to that. As we rolled out the plan, we did make mistakes in judgment about the people we promoted to leadership roles. Keep in mind that we are at early stages, so the turnover rate is reflecting small numbers. We are expecting to learn and do more as we continue.

Susan: I'm sorry to be blunt, Bob. It seems that at this stage, we have not done much but pay lip service to diversity. We need to be careful about glossing over the trouble spots because we could lose sight of one of our ultimate goals, which is to ensure that the composition of our leadership team reflects our diverse community. Although I applaud the efforts Mary and her team have already put in, more work is definitely needed. The program has to include specific plans and actions to boost diversity recruitment, retention, and promotion. If capable diverse candidates aren't being hired, then we aren't as great at finding candidates as we think we are. We need to reconsider our plan of action.

While this meeting heats up, another debate is sparking.

Margaret, the vice president of human resources at Alpha's flagship hospital, is amid a lengthy discussion with Wally, the chief information officer, and Dr. Masters, the chief medical officer. At issue is the decision to fill the position of chief medical information officer (CMIO). Both Wally and Dr. Masters favor the internal promotion of Dr. Johnson, who has practiced at the hospital for many years and has served as its chief of staff. However, Margaret sees the opening as an opportunity to hire a qualified, external, diverse candidate.

Margaret: Gentlemen, I agree that Dr. Johnson is well liked by the medical staff and is an astute observer of information technology trends. However, our search team has delivered to us two extremely qualified contenders. Dr. Backus has a master's in IT (information technology) and substantial experience in implementing electronic health records. Dr. Edmonds has been involved in IT planning and implementation for numerous years. Dr. Johnson, on the other hand, does not fully meet the qualifications listed in the job description. We interviewed him as a courtesy, but frankly he is not a viable candidate.

Dr. Masters: I agree that Dr. Backus and Dr. Edmonds have good qualifications for the role. But an outsider is going to be a risk, and it's one I'm not willing to take. In the coming months, the new CMIO will roll out major changes that will touch every clinical user. To make sure that this initiative is supported and successful, it needs a leader whom the medical staff can trust. That leader is Dr. Johnson. Wally agrees with me on this, and we are ready to make an offer to him.

THIS TWO-IN-ONE VIGNETTE touches on the different perceptions of diversity at multiple organizational and leadership levels. At the system and C-suite levels, the emphasis can be on program development and establishment of actionable goals. At the hospital and departmental levels, the focus often needs to be implementation. The vignette also poses a question that most, if not all, leaders grapple with at least once during their careers: What guides diversity hiring—the merits or capabilities of candidates, the goal of the organization to diversify its employee and leadership bases, or the personal preferences of the decision maker?

In this chapter, we explore the tensions faced by leaders from historically under-represented groups (e.g., racial minorities, women). Also, we suggest approaches for lending support to diverse leaders and learning about the realities of diversity. Our primary focus is on leaders from the majority group—male and Caucasian—who want to develop and support their under-represented leaders. Our decision to focus on this group is purposeful in that, at this time, the executive ranks in most healthcare organizations remain dominated by white men. Our presentation is informed by our experience and our discussions with diverse leaders.[1]

PRESSURES ON UNDER-REPRESENTED LEADERS

Healthcare leadership in the United States has a long history of being highly homogeneous. Many under-represented or diverse leaders sense a pressure to comply or fit into the majority or dominant group, or they may even hide or give up aspects of their personage that are representative of their diverse background. Examples of these efforts include talking or dressing in a manner similar to that of the majority group at work. In addition to these visible changes, many diverse leaders face less visible psychological challenges while pursuing their careers.

Establishing Legitimacy

Unlike their majority-group peers, leaders from diverse backgrounds may feel additional pressure to establish a sense of legitimacy within the profession. The drive to establish personal and professional legitimacy can have both positive and negative outcomes. On the positive side, the energy that diverse leaders pour into all their endeavors allows them to be noticed by superiors. They display interest, curiosity, willingness to help and participate, knowledge, and motivation, all of which indicate that they are equally as capable as their peers, if not more capable. As a result, they stand out from the rest because of their contributions, not their demographic difference.

The negative side of this tendency can be perfectionism—a need for every task and accomplishment to be a winner. The tendency can run against the leader as he ascends the organizational ladder. In higher-level positions, the leader needs to be comfortable with taking substantial risks, putting forward ideas and initiatives that may or may not succeed and then facing the consequences of both failures and successes. Taking bold stances is challenging even for leaders from the dominant group. It is particularly taxing for an under-represented leader, whose social capital (see Chapter 7) may not be as robust and who may fear being used as a scapegoat if the risky decision turns out to be a mistake.

Dealing with Isolation

It is indeed lonely at the top. For under-represented leaders, the isolation can be compounded by being among the first of their group to reach the institution's C-suite. Fortunately, a number of professional associations provide additional support for leaders in these circumstances. We recommend that you encourage your diverse leaders to participate; the benefits offered by these groups typically exceed the costs of membership. See the following section for a discussion on supporting your under-represented leaders.

SOURCES AND STRATEGIES FOR REACHING OUT AND LEARNING MORE

The first step to developing diverse talent is gaining an appreciation for the additional challenges these leaders face.

Develop Your Awareness

Awareness and understanding of diversity and leadership will equip you to have open discussions, to make decisions that are more considerate and appropriate, and to leverage diversity to provide the greatest outcomes. In addition, it will enable you to better guide a diverse workforce and will prevent you from committing common mistakes.

For example, well-meaning executives have mistakenly made a general assumption that their diverse leaders offer a specific "perspective" (e.g., the African-American perspective, the female perspective, or the Jewish perspective). In reality, many leaders from diverse backgrounds do not consider their views to be representative of their respective groups, and they resent being put in this position or pigeonholed. Developing a greater awareness is especially critical for executives who grew up in homogenous communities or who spent most of their careers in homogeneous organizations, as they likely have an underdeveloped sense of the dynamics of diversity in the workplace.

Offer Support

Many diverse leaders benefit most from having access to the additional professional and social supports their majority-group peers take for granted. Here are some strategies for supplying that support.

1. *Provide an opportunity to discuss the pressures faced by diverse leaders.* You do not have to be an expert on diversity issues, but you have to be aware of them. Send the message that you are open to and comfortable with addressing any challenges and barriers to success they may encounter.
2. *Be inclusive and accommodating.* This includes avoiding, as much as possible, holding critical meetings or events at times when these leaders are away from the office for professional or personal reasons. This simple act will communicate to the leader that you do not want to exclude him and that you value his presence and participation. The same approach should be followed for scheduling social activities, such as social outings or family-oriented events.
3. *Encourage active participation in professional associations,* such as the National Association of Health Services Executives (see www.nahse.org),[2] the National Forum of Latino Healthcare Executives (see www.nflhe.org), the Asian Health Care Leaders Association (see www.asianhealthcareleaders.org), and Women Health Executive Network (see www.whenchicago.org, for example). Healthcare organizations can also

communicate and make visible their support of diversity in leadership by getting involved with the Institute for Diversity in Health Management (see www.diversityconnection.org) or other workplace diversity efforts. Exposure to these networks will help both you and your under-represented direct reports gain an appreciation for the nuances of managing and developing diverse talents.

Immerse Yourself

Undergoing an immersive experience is an effective initial approach to diversity awareness. For example, a senior executive may volunteer to work for several months in an inner-city clinic, a women's shelter, or a refugee camp, in which he is the only white, Christian, American, English speaker. Over the course of his stay, the executive will reflect extensively, comparing and contrasting his own experiences and perspectives with those of the people he is helping. The inevitable result is a greater appreciation of others' circumstances, realities, and points of view.

Welcome Dialogues

You may establish a forum in which people can openly discuss diversity-related topics, such as similarities and differences in personal and professional experiences. While a tight structure is usually not necessary or helpful, a few ground rules for this forum can be helpful to ensure that it remains as focused, respectful, and informative as possible. Participants in these dialogues often find them to be an ideal launch pad for seeking out additional opportunities to learn about people whose backgrounds are different from their own.

APPLICATION TO THE C-SUITE

Healthcare organizations that have made the most progress toward the goal of diversifying the leadership team implemented three steps: (1) increased the communication about the importance of diversity, (2) assigned individual accountability to diverse hiring and retention functions, and (3) made the strategic development of high-potential diverse leaders a priority. Reflecting a long-term perspective, these institutions start early, identifying minority employees at various leadership levels as the targets for development.

Unfortunately, moving diverse leaders into the C-suite remains a formidable task in healthcare. The decline of fellowship and other rotational opportunities exacerbates these difficulties. C-suite leaders must do far more to open up their doors, including, at a minimum, discussing diversity on a regular basis, setting formal diversity goals and making individuals accountable for the results, and viewing diversity as a senior leadership, not a human resources, mandate.

NOTES

1. We reached out to several well-established leaders from diverse backgrounds to augment our own perspective, including Howard Jessamy, Oliver Tomlin, Judson Allen, Walter McLarty, Barbara Palmer, Steve Yamada, and Michelle Taylor-Smith. Their insights helped us shape this chapter.

2. As of this writing, NAHSE has about 24 active chapters across the United States. For chapter locations and contact information, go to the "Chapters" section on the NAHSE website.

CHAPTER 11

Mastering Differences in Age and Tenure

Juanita is a chief executive officer. At the airport, on her way home from a governance conference, she met two other attendees, Phil and Stella, both of whom are also senior leaders.

Juanita: Did you enjoy the sessions?

Stella: They were good, although I was amazed by the number of young people in the audience!

Juanita: I noticed that, too. They are probably still students or just graduated. I thought, Do these kids expect to just waltz right out of grad school and into the boardroom?

Phil: These young administrators have a completely different mind-set. They don't want to work beyond a straight eight, they can't learn anything on their own, and they have no concept of "paying your dues." About nine months ago, I hired this guy fresh out of school. Six months into his role, he was angling to be a director. I gave it to him straight: You don't even have one year under your belt, so you're nowhere near ready to be director. Did he listen? Heck no! He left to take another position for an administrator who didn't know any better.

Stella: I can relate. I experience the same things with nurse leadership. This new generation of workers wants it all. When I was rising up the ranks, the job's needs always came first. Nowadays, the only way to entice people into taking a management role is to convince them it will allow them more control over their schedule. Then, when they are finally on board, they don't take the position seriously, treating it as if it will always be there. The ambitious ones, on the other hand, are always at your door about a raise or a promotion.

Juanita: We certainly had different pressures a generation ago. I work with plenty of people who sacrificed their chance to have a family for the sake of having a career. Luckily, my daughter didn't follow this route. She got into a leadership role early in her career, and then took time off to start a family, something that was unheard of when I started my career. Now, she juggles multiple roles as a mother, a wife, and a vice president in a small hospital.

Phil: I must admit, though, that young people seem to adapt to change a lot better than we do. They also seem to be more productive and able to multitask, with the help of their "crackberries" and other gadgets. Those are important assets in healthcare, now more than ever.

THIS VIGNETTE RAISES a number of themes that are representative of today's workplace: perceived differences between younger and older leaders in work values, career expectations, and use of technology. In this chapter, we address these dynamics with a focus on how age and tenure shape our work views, attitudes, and priorities. These, in turn, should affect your approach to leadership development. Before anything else, however, a discussion about the "generation gap" is helpful in pinpointing the source of the differences in values and attitudes among leaders.

GENERATION GAP

In the modern work environment, the phrase "generation gap" has become an overused and oversimplified explanation of the distinction between new and long-term careerists. Originally, the term highlighted the generational divide between parents and children in the backdrop of historical or cultural events that marked a given period or generation, such as the assassinations of John F. Kennedy and Martin Luther King Jr. and the terrorist attacks on September 11, 2001. These kinds of events have varying degrees of impact, depending on the person's age and experience at the time they occurred. For example, a discussion of the Vietnam War will elicit a much stronger response from baby boomers than among generation Xers. The question is whether these events significantly change a person's approach to leadership, fundamental personality, or value system.

In terms of the workplace, how do generation differences influence an employee's performance and values and her opinions of those she deems unlike her? Is an older worker more loyal and accountable? Does a younger staff member care only about his own interests? According to findings of a research study involving almost 1,300 leaders, the differences are not as large as one may think (see Figure 11.1 for the complete results). Respondents in this survey, regardless of their age, cited the same need for trust and respect and the same dislike for change. Most of the differences attributed to generation gaps were found to be the functions of life stages, experiences, or job levels, not generational traits. That is, the younger generation is not less loyal to their organization, but they are more "willing to move" to progress in their careers. Baby boomers, on the other hand, do not relish working long hours; they do so because it is an expectation of their senior-level jobs.

If the so-called generation gap is not the reason that your values are different from those of your leaders, particularly your junior associates, then what is behind these differences? Chalk it up to a difference in perspective, not generations. We all tend to use ourselves (and those similar to us) as the primary reference point for everything we experience. This is a natural tendency, a default way of understanding how our experiences and perspectives fit with those of others, and vice versa. This is why age and tenure drive our differences more than our generation gap does.

Figure 11.1 Research Suggests More Commonalities than Differences Across Generations of Leaders

Are there generational differences in leaders? Research involving approximately 1,300 leaders suggests an overlap more than a gap. Here are some of the many similarities this work revealed.

- *We have similar values.* Although expressed differently, these values are prioritized the same way across generations. "Family" always gets top billing, and "integrity" is not far behind. In contrast, "achievement" is relatively low on the list.
- *We want respect.* The definition of respect depends on leaders' position levels, which can make it seem like a generational difference. At lower levels, respect is viewed as the ability to have a voice in the process, while at higher levels, respect involves the recognition that the leader's opinion is worthy because it is informed by experience.
- *We value trust.* Every leader, regardless of age or tenure, places a high premium on openness, honesty, and transparency. Also, they all trust people with whom they have worked more than they trust those they have not worked with.
- *We are loyal.* Although younger leaders are more likely to job-hop, they do not do so any more frequently than the prior generations of leaders did at the beginning of their careers. Similarly, they do not work less than their older peers. In fact, the average number of hours worked per week is heavily influenced by the leader's position level, not age.
- *We do not like change.* Despite the folk wisdom that older people are more resistant to change, the reality is all leaders struggle in the face of change. Aversion or attraction to change is not a product of age differences; it is related to the individual's hopes, fears, and tendency toward stability and predictability.
- *We want to learn.* The presence or lack of opportunities for learning has an enormous influence on job satisfaction. This is true regardless of the leader's age or generation.

Source: Information from Deal (2007).

IMPACT OF AGE ON WORK RELATIONSHIPS

Discrimination based on age (for employees aged 40 or older) is forbidden under the Age Discrimination in Employment Act. This law has caused some amount of caution in the workplace, particularly in the context of hiring and promotion. However, in the context of forging better work relationships and for the purpose of understanding leadership development, age remains an important factor. In this section, we explore the two age categories in leadership that may cause tensions among the team.

Younger Leader

At a young age, most of us learned to show respect and deference to older people. Conversely, we learned to expect respect and deference from younger individuals. This is a straightforward, beneficial practice in polite society. However, this same approach can be complicated in leadership, where exceptional performance may lead to a senior-level position at a young age.

When a leader is significantly younger than his peers or direct reports, conflict may be inevitable. The following are some common reactions to this age gap:

- *Jealousy.* Direct reports, and even peers, who are frustrated by their own career trajectories may harbor envy for the younger leader. Such resentment may manifest in unspoken but visible hostility and even outright sabotage.
- *Intimidation.* A leader's rapid rise to the C-suite may intimidate her direct reports. They may view her as so infallible as to have achieved so much in such a short time. As a result, they defer to her decisions all the time, reluctant to share their views and knowledge, preventing the level of learning that the new leader needs to succeed.

- *Fear.* Older workers, particularly those who do not feel secure in their own roles, may view the leader with a degree of suspicion. For example, a simple question from the leader about an employee's tenure may trigger anxiety about staff reductions. At a deeper level, older employees may view the young leader as the embodiment of their fear that their own tenure with the organization is coming to an end.

Addressing leadership problems. In coaching a younger leader, you can introduce the topic of age relatively safely by stating the obvious: "Joe is a lot older than you. That kind of age gap can create conflicts in a reporting relationship. How are you two getting along?" From there, encourage the leader to be honest about the challenges she has experienced pertaining to the age difference. Offer your perspective on the situation and on the leader's direct reports. This insight may help the leader better understand her staff's behavior.

If the leader is trying to change her staff's attitude toward her, encourage her to concentrate on building a relationship with each of them. A good place to start is to have a one-on-one conversation with each of her staff. A particularly skillful leader may be able to put the subject of age directly on the table through a role-modeling opening such as, "I have to confess: It's a new experience for me to be in a supervisory relationship with someone who has so many more years of experience than I do. And I also wonder what you think about our differences."

These conversations can open the door to better communication, which, in turn, can become a basis for trust. However, such dialogues do not work in all circumstances. Sometimes, a direct report, or even a peer, cannot overcome his initial response or prejudice enough to allow a productive working relationship. In these cases, the leader has to either work around the person (if a peer) or redeploy or counsel him (if a direct report). This decision must be always driven by the person's underperformance, not his attitude about the age difference.

Older Leader

Leaders who are significantly older (20 or more years) than their peers or employees also run into challenges. For example, they may tend to underestimate the amount of time and effort needed by a newcomer to "learn the ropes" or reach a minimally acceptable level of productivity in the department or the organization. Also, older leaders who are at or near the end of their career may not relate well to direct reports who are just beginning theirs. These leaders may fail to recognize and appropriately channel the early careerists' energy and ambition.

Addressing leadership problems. The clearest signal that the older leader may not be in touch with the needs of his younger staff is an unusually high turnover rate in his department. You can help this leader by finding out if the needs of his younger staff are clear to him. First, ask about his staff's career goals and ambitions. If the leader has a good grasp of these goals, ask what he is doing to support their development. Often, such a leader can benefit the most from developing his skills in mentoring younger leaders, including delegating more.

With a little help, many older executives can become outstanding mentors. As they enter a more reflective period in life, they may find tremendous personal fulfillment in helping up-and-comers sort out their career interests and plans. In addition, these leaders may be valuable resources in leadership development or talent management programs.

Employment attorneys routinely warn individuals **not** to discuss age with older workers. If the older worker loses a chance for promotion or loses his position, the discussion may become prima facie evidence of age discrimination. Openness and honesty are generally the best policy. However, in this area an open discussion may be more a liability than an asset.

INFLUENCE OF TENURE

Tenure is the length of time a person has worked in a given job or organization. Two kinds of tenure are common in healthcare organizations: lifers and long-tenure roles.

"Lifers"

Lifers are the organization's long-term employees. They are the backbone of the organization, providing stable and reliable service and even shaping the culture. Many such employees develop deep ties with the organization, and through their long tenures come to enjoy a comfortable, rewarding workplace.

This comfort can also create an aversion to change, which can be both helpful and harmful to the organization's development: helpful in that it prevents half-baked ideas from being implemented, and harmful in that it slows down (or prevents) badly needed changes from taking place.

When first coming in to an organization, this "backbone" against and around which change must be implemented is nearly invisible. Newly hired leaders must invest the time to get to know the lifer dynamics before rolling out any grand plan. Otherwise, direct opposition, in the form of missed deadlines and other disruptions, may occur.

Long-Tenure Roles

Long-tenure roles involve employees who have filled the same specific position, particularly a leadership role, for many years or even decades. Like a lifer, a long-term professional typically delivers reliable performance and outcomes.

The danger of long-tenure roles is that job performance becomes increasingly habit driven. The tendency to do things the same way grows, and opportunities for improvement are overlooked.

You can help prevent stagnation in long-tenure roles by reviewing jobs against job descriptions every several years. Ideally, every role will see at least some growth and evolution during that period, and the descriptions can be adjusted accordingly. If no such growth has occurred in at least five years, you should proactively seek ways to develop, expand, or add new challenges to the role (see Chapter 4 for examples).

Job rotation is another way to help minimize the possibility of stagnation. Job rotation can be used for special projects or for longer-term (greater than six months) assignments in another department or area.

Initially, the leader may resist such changes. However, they serve to keep the leader conscious of his duties and continually developing his skills. At the least, you should set clear performance benchmarks so that expectations for continuous performance improvement are being clearly communicated and encouraged.

APPLICATION TO THE C-SUITE

Many C-suites are made up of leaders who are in the same age range and who have served in the organization (or another) for a similar length of time. Amazingly, a close look at the senior leadership teams of many healthcare organizations shows a significant sameness in age and experiences. Age and tenure may communicate that the leadership team has solid experience and stability, but at times, a lack of fresh perspective from younger and newer executives can lead to groupthink. A senior leadership team that stays the same for years can also signal that the team does not welcome junior members and thus the only hope for promotion to the C-suite is to either stay on for a long time or leave the organization for an opportunity elsewhere.

To avoid this potential problem, senior teams can try the following:

- Use post-graduate fellowship programs to ensure the presence of a "new face" in the senior leadership ranks. Fellows are often welcome to ask questions and to challenge how and why certain decisions are made.
- On a rotating basis, invite a department manager to sit in on senior team meetings. The dynamic of the meetings will often change, and the opportunity for exposure will enhance the growth potential of the department manager. Many executives use this approach to broaden their senior-team thinking and increase middle management's understanding of the role of senior management.
- Use middle managers to lead special task forces even when senior managers will be represented on these groups.

REFERENCE

Deal, J. J. 2007. *Retiring the Generation Gap: How Employees Young and Old Can Find Common Ground.* San Francisco: Jossey-Bass.

Handling Delicate Transitions

For several years now, Dr. Ali, a member of the medical staff at a community hospital, has been thinking of a move to an administrative role. He finds that his clinical practice is no longer rewarding, and his recent involvement with the quality committee at the hospital and his service as a member-at-large on the medical executive committee only fueled his interest in management. As soon as the associate vice president of medical affairs position became vacant, Dr. Ali approached Dr. Anderson, the vice president of medical affairs, to discuss the possibility of his move.

Dr. Anderson: Why do you think you want this job?

Dr. Ali: I've been in a clinical role for more than ten years, and I'm ready for a change. The call coverage in the last two years has been particularly rough; I'd like to see the middle-of-the-night phone calls happen a lot less frequently. A management position would also offer a more stable income, which will be helpful as my kids are almost college-aged. But money is not my main driver. Based on my experience and accomplishments with the performance improvement committee and the quality task force, I think I have a knack for management.

Dr. Anderson: Tell me more about what you like about management itself.

Dr. Ali: I certainly enjoyed the projects. It was a privilege to work with a diverse group of doctors, executives, and staff.

Dr. Anderson: What questions can I answer for you?

Dr. Ali: I'd like to know your vision for the associate vice president position. Then, I want to know if I am qualified, and if not what improvements I can make to my existing skills.

Dr. Anderson: I'm not sure that we're ready for that conversation yet.

Dr. Ali: I don't understand. I came under the impression that you and I can candidly discuss this matter. What are we ready to talk about?

Dr. Anderson: I understand that you have thought through your decision to move away from clinical work. But I am not yet convinced that you have thought through a move into management. I will be candid with you now: Making a transition from clinical to administrative work involves so much more than sporadic involvement with task forces and committees. There are advantages, but also drawbacks and dangers that go with them. Before talking about this specific position, I need more confidence that you know what you are getting yourself into, both professionally and personally. After our discussion, you need to take some time to ponder if this is really the route you want to take.

AS THIS VIGNETTE illustrates, a transition from a clinical to a managerial post can appear deceptively straightforward. In reality, this is one of the most profound shifts in the healthcare leadership profession. Not only does it require major time investments and reprioritization, but it also demands a substantial change in professional identity, career plans, and even social relationships. For these and other reasons, this transition is often difficult to navigate successfully.

We use the phrase "delicate transition" to indicate the need for tactful and careful handling of such moves. In this chapter, typical changes experienced in three common leadership transitions that tend to be delicate are explained: (1) changes that occur when one moves from clinician to leader, (2) changes that accompany promotions involving major expansions of responsibility, and (3) changes that result from moves into and within the C-suite. Along the way, we offer insights on helping you or your leaders handle these transitions most effectively.

FROM CLINICIAN TO LEADER

Clinicians complete extensive, often lengthy training to become highly skilled providers of patient care. Many clinical professions—nursing and medicine in particular—have strong professional identities, which young people may feel "called to" at a relatively early age. For these clinicians, their work is as much who they are as what they do.

Advocacy on behalf of their patients is often a key part of this professional identity. Many clinicians regard organizational leaders with suspicion, feeling that they should be perpetually on guard for management's seemingly continuous parade of intrusions into their professional autonomy. Thus, a transition to a leadership role often involves an unforeseen renegotiation of identity.

Unexpected Changes

One main concern for clinicians is that they feel caught between the needs of their patients and the limits set by the organization. A lot of clinicians intend, at least in part, to move into leadership roles to have greater influence over patient care. They may feel they are pursuing the new role with "open eyes," particularly if they have already gained experience with committee and project-based work that has exposed them to the multiple administrative challenges and conflicts. Once ensconced in the position, however, they experience unexpected consequences of their transition, such as the following:

- *Diminished opportunities for direct patient contact.* Even physicians and nurses who left clinical practice because they felt fatigued or burned out may find they miss direct patient care. In their leadership roles, their patient contact may be focused primarily on addressing service failures (e.g., responding to the frustrations of patients and their families, or investigating system failures that have caused patients harm). In these cases, finding opportunities to reconnect with the positive sides of patient care can be helpful to clinicians as they adjust to their new roles—for example, roles involving philanthropy, public relations, community outreach, or customer service recognition programs.

- *Change in social support.* Leaders need to be objective decision makers, acting as agents on behalf of the mission of their organizations. For this reason, many clinicians-turned-leaders find they need to distance themselves from the clinicians who once served as their primary source of social support. They no longer have the frequent interaction with clinical peers in treatment areas, and they find that they actually develop broader perspectives about organizational strategies and priorities. In turn, for many of the same reasons, their clinical peers tend to regard the new leader with suspicion or even hostility. The common phrase used in healthcare is that the clinician "has now gone over to the dark side." Discussing and reflecting on this change can be beneficial for the clinician leader. Helping or encouraging him to form relationships with other clinician leaders and colleagues can also ease the initial social loss inherent in the transition experience.

- *Loss of professional identity.* Professional identity helps a clinician feel that she has a professional "home" and that her work contributes to a broader purpose. A transition to management, which provides few chances for direct patient care and alters the former clinician's social circle, can make the new leader feel as if she is an outsider in her own profession. This feeling is especially intense in academic medical settings, which may require the clinician leader to give up her preceptor role, other ties to clinical education, or regular attendance at professional conferences, where long-standing collegial ties used to be refreshed. You can help clinician leaders cope with this loss by encouraging them to embrace a new professional identity as a healthcare executive. Introducing them to relevant professional associations and trade groups, even offering to attend a conference with them, can ease these transitions.

Changes Specific to Physician and Nurse Leaders

Nurses. In many healthcare organizations, nurses interested in career advancement must choose between two paths: (1) increased clinical expertise and (2) increased management responsibility. The clinical track is often considered to be more prestigious and more closely tied to the mission of the profession. This perception is unfortunate because it dissuades many talented potential nurse leaders from giving the management track a chance.

Organizations with strong nursing leadership overcome these challenges by placing greater emphasis on these career tracks—through internal leadership development programs, formal succession planning, and greater emphasis on having nurses "at the table" for important decisions.

Nurses who transition into management roles tend to bring interpersonal and clinical expertise as a result of their academic and practical training, but typically also need skill development in traditional management areas such as accounting, finance, and human resource management, which are rarely covered in clinical programs.

Physicians. Typically, physicians enter into leadership roles with both intellectual and persuasive communications horsepower. This combination can mask important deficits in experience with key management areas such as finance, operations, and marketing. Because most physicians are accustomed to reaching clear clinical decisions, many who become leaders are initially perplexed by the myriad ambiguous guidelines for management decision making.

Many also find they need to tune their interpersonal skills, which are essential to executive-level positions.

Fortunately, most physicians are quick studies, and are able to master these skills through executive education programs. As a chief leader, you may guide their learning with carefully chosen project assignments and on-the-job exposures to management principles. Mentors in appropriate functional areas are also helpful in this regard.

The nature of the physician's employment is altered when she becomes an executive. In clinical practice, physician income may vary but employment is highly secure, except in the event of a serious ethical breach or a malpractice case. Leadership, in contrast, offers a steady salary but within at-will employment; as such, the physician executive can lose his job with little notice or recourse. In addition, the starting salary for a physician leader may be substantially lower than the income for a specialist. This pay difference is one of the reasons physician leadership roles tend to be filled by primary care doctors.

In transitioning to management, the physician's approach will shift:

- *From patient advocate to organization advocate.* In an ideal world, these two goals would never be mutually exclusive. In reality, however, the physician executive must act in the best interests of the organization, which are not always aligned with the needs of individual patients or the clinicians caring for them.
- *From short-term to long-term time frames.* As one physician leader aptly put it, "I realized when I became a vice president of medical affairs that I had moved from dealing in ten-minute increments to year-long increments." Physician executives no longer get to provide the immediate fixes, services, or treatments they did during their clinical roles; instead, they operate under long-term strategies and plans.

Finally, encourage your physician leaders to avoid using the derogatory (even if meant as a joke) phrase, "moved to the dark side." They should also prepare a positive response when confronted with this remark, and in general should emphasize the importance of collaboration.

MAJOR PROMOTION

In Chapter 3, we argue that a move from one career stage to another (i.e., a major promotion) requires a change in approach and a renegotiation of relationships. In this section, we apply that idea to the transition following a promotion.

Change in Approach

Leaders ascending a career stage will face new realities at the leadership level, including the following:

- *Limited physical interaction with direct reports.* At the executive level, direct reports typically do not share the same physical area with their superiors. The new leader, who may be used to meeting with her former staff several times per day, will need to find a new approach to keeping communication lines open with her group.
- *Long-term emphasis.* The majority of a department manager's work, such as budgeting and performance review, is based on annual cycles. Work at the executive level, such as strategic planning, involves a multicycle time horizon. The promoted leader, then, has to think in terms of future scenarios, considering multiple possibilities and synthesizing them into a general contingency plan.
- *Coalition building.* In comparison to middle and department managers, the lines of authority at the executive level are

less clear. As a result, executives must work to balance their accountabilities to multiple individuals. Success at this level requires the executive to lead more through influence than authority, engaging in building relationships without appearing too political. The leader needs to be candid and direct, not play favorites, and recognize the rules of reciprocity or pay back.

- *Broad perspective.* The new executive's loyalty must be to the organization as a whole, not to any particular department or area. If a leader's focus is too narrow, it will result in animosity and infighting within the team and may weaken newly forged relationships with peers. The role of peer support in the success of the leader is also heightened significantly at the executive level.

Renegotiation of Relationships

After the leader's transition, some of his former peers will want to maintain the same kind of close association they once had because doing so can afford them influence. Meanwhile, some new colleagues will not immediately accept the legitimacy of the leader's promotion and will withhold their support. As the latest addition to the leadership team, the executive often must work harder to ensure he is in the loop about important meetings and is receiving relevant communications from his peers.

The executive should set parameters for continuing his relationship with former peers. This can be done most efficiently through individual meetings to discuss how the nature of the working relationship will change. In terms of his new colleagues, early on the leader should identify one or two other executives on the team who can serve as guides, helping him understand the history and culture of the group as well as each member's styles and preferences. The new leader's superior or senior human resource executives can also help in this part of the on-boarding.

INTO AND WITHIN THE C-SUITE

This section presents the dynamics at play behind the proverbial "mahogany doors," which can include all of the challenges previously discussed as well as a number of new ones.

Into the C-Suite

For many healthcare administrators, the transition into the C-suite is the most exciting step of their careers. It is an enormous, often daunting, step forward that presents several new transitional challenges, including the following:

Acceptance by mid-level managers. A leader who was promoted from within often has an easier time gaining acceptance by middle management, who will regard that person as "one of our own." The history of working relationships is also an asset to both the promoted leader and the mid-level managers. Middle managers are often not as supportive of a leader who was brought in from another organization. This executive may find herself challenged most of the time, particularly when she pushes for rapid changes that conflict with the established practices and procedures. In extreme cases, the managers may draw their power together to oppose the leader, substantially undermining her influence and effectiveness.

Difficult decisions. C-suite executives regularly make difficult, high-stakes decisions concerning the ideal allocation of limited resources in the face of competing needs. They need to stick to the mission and their own analyses to guide these decisions, despite the insistent and loud advocacy of many parties for their own causes. In their roles as agents of the organization, they may also be called on to adjudicate inter-departmental conflicts.

Shift from director to coordinator. According to first-time C-suite members we have talked to, the biggest difference they face is that they no longer feel directly involved in the hospital's day-to-day activities. The role of the C-suite executive is that of coordinator, not director. In this way, the leader is an extension of the CEO, overseeing a broader area rather than representing a particular part of the organization.

Within the C-Suite

Following are tricky challenges associated with a move within the C-suite.

From VP to COO. A peer-to-superior move can be complicated for several reasons. First, the selection of one VP over another may cause hard feelings and interpersonal tensions among members of senior management. Consequently, the VP who was passed over may plan to leave, believing that she has no future in the organization.

Second, the new COO's former collegial relationships may influence or hinder his decisions. The COO must set his agenda without deferring to the opinions and interests of his former peers.

Third, if a new COO does not have a clinical background, he will likely be challenged by VPs who do. The COO can respond to this opposition by taking seriously his need to develop a working knowledge of his VPs' clinical areas. He will also need to learn when to listen to these challenges and when to shrug them off.

Fourth, as a former VP, the COO may fall back to his old mode of directly approaching the department directors or managers when a problem arises. The COO needs to resist this impulse, instead allowing the VPs to represent their own areas.

From CNO to COO. The nursing profession is the largest employee base in any hospital, and its work has the most substantial impact on patient perceptions and satisfaction. Often, nursing's wide reach is envied and even resented by other clinical ("ancillary") and nonclinical groups. These negative feelings can carry over when a CNO is promoted to the C-suite.

A CNO recently promoted to the COO or CEO post may still identify strongly with her former area, making it difficult to give up the reins to the new CNO. Although some transition period may be anticipated in the beginning, any attempts for the former CNO to maintain control over time need to be addressed swiftly, so that her full attention is focused on her new role as quickly as possible.

To CEO. Most CEOs describe the role as impossible to fully prepare for; you only learn and master the CEO role on the job. The following realities of a healthcare CEO demand different approaches, no matter the previous position of the person who fills the role:

- *Multiple superiors.* The CEO of a not-for-profit hospital reports to a board, whose membership numbers from 5 to 25 or more community, business, and industry leaders. With this number comes diversity in personal background and traits, working styles and preferences, and leadership vision. In addition, a board's composition changes over time, which requires the CEO to face a new set of bosses with differing and sometimes conflicting agendas.
- *External stakeholders.* A CEO's success is tied to the success of his organization. The definition of this success goes beyond the achievement of outstanding performance or the accomplishment of goals. It also entails the positive reputation of the enterprise. The CEO needs to invest time building and managing relationships with the board and the surrounding community.
- *Visionary, not executor.* The CEO is at the center of crafting the organizational vision, but not the implementation of that vision. Many CEOs may regard this reality as having

less influence and control over the outcomes. However, the CEO does exert power by establishing the underlying vision and strategies. In the end, the CEO's performance is judged primarily on what results were achieved, not how they were accomplished.

- *Where the buck stops.* The CEO is ultimately responsible for everything that happens in or to the organization. As the head steward, she makes the final, often difficult, calls, with careful consideration of her leadership team's and the board's recommendations.

- *Public image.* Because the CEO is the face of the organization, his comments, both formal and informal, are sought after, meticulously scrutinized, and sometimes erroneously interpreted. A savvy CEO knows to wisely use public relations resources and to carefully monitor his image and his communications in public. He is aware that a remark such as "we are thinking about pursuing this initiative" can be misprinted or misquoted as "we will pursue this initiative." Even a simple expression of agreement can be taken out of context.

- *Filtered information.* Typically, the CEO receives only "final" information. All the planning, fact-finding, recommendations, deliberations, and iterations that went into the finished product have been removed. Without the backstory, much of this information must be taken on faith by the CEO, who must trust that his leadership team exercised due diligence.

  The carefully packaged information may be more convenient, but it could also be misleading. For example, explanation notes about numbers and figures may have a positive spin so as not to alarm or concern the CEO. Wise CEOs are vigilant for this phenomenon. They test the veracity of the reports by posing difficult questions, challenging the numbers, and requesting supporting documents. Also, they do not tolerate false or inaccurate presentation of information, but also cautiously avoid "killing the messenger" for telling it like it is.

- *Inadequate or missing feedback.* A CEO often does not get good feedback or hear disagreements and dissents. She may no longer be able to count on her colleagues to "tell it like it is," or to give her push-back when her plans or requests seem unreasonable. As a result, she can feel as if she is never wrong, and her ego can easily get overinflated. Even chief leaders who are well balanced, mature, accessible, and down to earth can start to "believe their own press releases" if they are not cautious.

- *Loneliness at the top.* The CEO is barraged with many personal and professional requests and proposals. In response, he must carefully manage his associations, ensuring that his ties are strictly professional and do not turn into conflicts of interest. The downside to being in this position is that the CEO must be cautious about considering anyone he works with to be a confidante or a friend.

From CEO to. . . . Given the unique nature of the CEO role, leaving the position is often extremely difficult. This is particularly true when the CEO is forced to leave her position and move into a lower-level leadership role. She will find it difficult to adjust and may end up managing as though she is the head executive in charge. In this case, she may either be reprimanded by the CEO or be forced out of the leadership role. Others regard their non-CEO posts as a "holding pattern," where they will wait until another CEO position becomes available.

CEOs who retire from the role also face transition challenges. Boards may be tempted to keep a retiring CEO around in some type of "consultative" role while the new CEO is learning the ropes or, worse, as a member of the board. Such a move is highly risky because it will undermine the authority of the new CEO. The new CEO needs full latitude, which is impossible when the previous CEO still wields influence. It is often far better for the retiring CEO to identify other ways he can contribute his talents outside the organization he has retired from.

CHAPTER 13

Pursuing Personal Development

Rich is a professor and chair of the master in health services administration program at a large university in the Midwest. Over the years, he has helped many of his former students launch their careers and then continue on to fill senior-level positions. He has also served as a mentor to many of these students along the way.

Michael, whom Rich has known for more than 15 years—first as a student and then as a fast-rising administrator—recently contacted Rich for insight about a CEO position he was pursuing. As always, Rich offered well-thought-out advice, urging Michael to weigh the pros and cons of the role. Several weeks later, they met again at an alumni event. Although Michael looked pleased to see his old friend, he appeared out of his element.

Rich: I don't mean to be intrusive, but you seem down. Anything we can talk about?

Michael: You always could read me like a book. It's about the CEO job we discussed not too long ago. And about other things. Maybe we should talk some time.

Rich: Why don't we talk now? This sounds important enough not to put off. I can catch up with the other alumni later this evening.

Michael: Okay, here goes. The system offered me the job last Friday.

Rich: Seems like that would be great news. There's more to the story?

Michael: You got me again. The package is truly generous, and the opportunity is too good to pass up. But I took your advice to heart and stalled them, instead of taking the offer on the spot. I had to consult with Linda first, because like I told you, the job would entail another move for her and the kids.

Rich: Linda's reaction wasn't what you were expecting?

Michael: You know, for years she had been my strongest supporter, encouraging and patient, taking a lot of the household and family load off me so I could focus on the career. But for the past several years, maybe the last five, she has complained more and more. She used to be proud of the volunteer work I did; now she challenges me constantly about it: Why do I need to do it, and why can't I just do the main job I'm paid to do? She almost never comes to events anymore. I'd tell her I need her there, and that used to sway her, but she has started saying she doesn't care.

Rich: I'm sorry to hear that, Michael. How did she react to the CEO news?

Michael: When I first told her about applying, she simply said, "fine." I didn't press harder for her opinion because I knew she would have put her foot down if she didn't agree. I went through the grueling interview process, and she acted indifferent the whole time. When the offer came, I immediately called her. I explained that this was the goal we had been working hard toward all these years.

Rich: What did she say?

Michael: She said, "Michael, if you take that job, you'd better be prepared to move alone."

THIS VIGNETTE DEPICTS only one of the many personal tensions and sacrifices faced by most healthcare executives and their loved ones. While some leaders work through these inevitable conflicts, ultimately being rewarded with their partners' greater support and understanding, others try to ignore the tensions, minimize them, or blame their partner for them. The consequences can range from perpetual tension to permanently damaged relationships.

Maintaining an effective integration of work and life pursuits involves constant negotiation. Unfortunately, few graduate programs, leadership seminars, and competency models address this issue, primarily because the personal is mistakenly regarded as a "nuisance factor," a reality of executive life but largely irrelevant to work performance. Research, however, clearly indicates otherwise, as we present in this chapter.

Our experience in management and working with leaders has convinced us that personal health and development are a critical foundation to professional growth and effectiveness. This chapter, the conclusion to this book, provides a head-on treatment of this topic: why it is important and how to incorporate it into the development of your leaders, as well as your own.

THE INFLUENCE OF WORK ON LIFE

Healthcare executives spend more time in the workplace than anywhere else. This reality alone means that experiences in the workplace tend to affect a leader's adult development more than any other influences. These effects are difficult to see on a daily basis. Any given decision, conversation, or relationship on the job may not have a substantial impact, but taken collectively and over time they can change the leader substantially.

This is the backdrop of leadership development. If your emphasis, as a chief leader, is strictly on the professional—quality improvement, outcomes achievement, and strategic performance—you are sending the message that the personal is really not important. Your leaders, hearing that message loudly and clearly, may in turn regard their personal growth as inconsequential in their preparation for greater roles and responsibilities. This would be a mistake, as the following findings suggest.

Research Findings

The following studies support a link between personal health and development and professional performance.

Exercise. Research by the Center for Creative Leadership documents that executives who exercise regularly are rated higher than their peers on leadership effectiveness (*HR Magazine* 2006). Exercise is an essential health maintenance activity, and its benefits extend beyond a stronger body. During a workout, the brain is disengaged from the normal to-do list, allowing the person to gain perspective about his tasks. Leaders who exercise regularly often report that they use their workout period productively—solving problems and planning (McDowell-Larsen 2006). A study of small-business owners reveals that many find they come up with their best ideas while exercising or doing other down-time activities (American Express 2007).

Self-concept. Self-concept refers to a leader's level of comfort with himself and his place in the world. In *Exceptional Leadership,* we cited research that links a leader's healthy self-concept to better job performance, openness to feedback and mentoring, and effective pursuit of strategic opportunities (Dye and Garman 2006). According to a study by Rode (2004), a strong relationship exists between self-concept and both work and life satisfaction. In other words, the most promising pathway to improving work and life satisfaction is not finding the right job or even the ideal living arrangements, but rather in having greater comfort with oneself.

Self-awareness. In a work context, self-awareness is the extent to which a leader's self-appraisal of her strengths and development needs agrees with the appraisal her direct reports give her. Research indicates that high-performing managers are significantly more self-aware than their peers (Church 1997). Leaders can improve their self-awareness by listening to, and reflecting on, the opinions of those they work with (Wilson and Dunn 2004).

Disciplined practice. Learning to become a superb leader may be compared to training to become a better athlete or practicing to become a better musician. The rigorous discipline required of athletes and artists can also apply to executives. That is, a leader should master her "inner game," maintain her physical and mental health, and allow for periods of rest and recovery after exerting intense focus and energy.

Time away from the job. The United States is well known as a country where little vacation time is given and taken. What gets less attention is the clear benefits that vacations provide—benefits that we miss out on when we forgo these breaks. Research indicates that vacations reduce stress and job burnout (Westman and Eden 1997). They also improve people's health: Men at risk for coronary heart disease who do not take annual vacations have a 21 percent higher risk of death from all causes and are 32 percent more likely to die from a heart attack (Gump and Matthews 2000).

STRATEGIES FOR SUPPORTING PERSONAL GROWTH AND RENEWAL

Helping your leaders develop effective personal habits is as much about setting the right tone as giving advice or directives. Here are some steps to set the right tone.

Validate the Need

Do not underestimate the value of talking about the importance of personal growth, reflection, and renewal. These pursuits are more than abstract virtues; they are an essential part of becoming a more effective leader. A centered and balanced leader is someone who will be easier for others to trust, to follow, and to go the extra mile for.

Share Your Own Experiences

Think of times in your career when personal reflection led you to change course for the better. The catalyst may have been a discussion with your significant other, a trusted colleague, a mentor, or a direct superior. Sharing your own insights, and how you got to them, can be an incredibly powerful endorsement for the value of reflection and the importance of attending to personal growth.

Encourage "Unplugging"

Leaders need to disengage from the workplace from time to time. Time away from the regular routine, regardless of the length, gives leaders the opportunity to gain perspective on areas where the velocity of decisions may exceed the time available to think. Because of wireless and remote-access technology, however, "unplugging" from work-related e-mail, text, and voicemail messages has become a willful, rather than a natural, act.

If your leaders are reluctant or uncomfortable with occasionally going unplugged, try the following:

- *Convey that leaders need time to reflect.* A leader who stays plugged in at all times may not realize that time for reflection and renewal will benefit them and, by extension, their work. They may either think everyone works the same way they do or that everyone should. Labeling this "always-on" behavior as problematic may at first seem counterintuitive (isn't it handier to always have access to our leaders?). But this is an important start to a conversation about whether staying always plugged in benefits them and their organization as much as they think.
- *Probe the reasons for always being in touch.* Some leaders stay accessible because they do not want to "abandon" their staff and peers, while others fear that the walls may literally crash

down if they are not around. Often, there is an underlying explanation for these fears. Lack of faith in direct reports may be one of them. As leaders need to earn the trust of their direct reports, so too must direct reports build the trust of their leaders. Executives must give their staff a chance to cultivate this trust, allowing their employees to take the reins sometimes and, by doing so, expand their responsibilities.

- *Make an emergency-access arrangement.* Emergencies that need the input or intervention of the leader do arise, but they should not prevent her from taking time off for reflection. A good solution is to create an emergency plan, where the leader can be reached (at a phone number she prefers) only in a case of dire need. An even better strategy is to assign one of the leader's direct reports as the person in charge while she is out. The interim then keeps the leader's emergency contact number, makes the decision on what constitutes an emergency, and calls the leader if necessary.

Respect the Life Behind the Work

Healthcare executives give so much to their demanding jobs. They deserve respect not only for their contributions but also for having the sense to set limits to take care of their personal needs. As other professionals do, many executives strain to maintain satisfactory attendance and performance on the job while grappling with life's challenges. High-performing leaders especially have a difficult time asking for help or taking a break to tend to their life outside of work.

An offer to a struggling leader to take time off will indicate your support and concern for the leader's welfare. This simple move will immediately relieve some of his work stresses and will pay substantial dividends when he returns. The following is an example of how a proactive CEO handled a situation in which an executive's work and familial responsibilities were coming into increasing conflict.

Alina, an exemplary healthcare executive, is the daughter of elderly parents. Although her parents still lived independently—an arrangement they desperately wanted to maintain—over time, this arrangement was requiring Alina to step in more and more to help. For many months, Alina's everyday schedule was arduous: During the day, she worked at the hospital for at least ten hours, and at night, she rushed to her parents' house to take care of their needs. She remained productive on the job, but her physical, mental, and emotional strain was becoming visible to her staff and colleagues.

One day, John, her superior, pulled her into his office and diplomatically expressed his concerns. She told him about the extra strain of her parents' deteriorating functioning, and John appreciated her desire to help her parents maintain their home and independence. John disclosed that he could relate to her dilemma, as he went through a similar situation. He shared his difficulty with taking care of his mother and with telling her that she had to move into an assisted living facility, a step that turned out to be the best for everyone involved.

John told Alina he wanted to help her. She asked for his insights and suggestions, and the two of them weighed the pros and cons of each option. In the end, Alina settled on a solution that involved a leave of absence, allowing her to dedicate herself fully to having a heart-to-heart conversation with her parents and then finding a more workable living arrangement for them.

Alina's extended leave was tough on her department generally, and John in particular. But everyone managed well enough. When Alina returned, she was more energetic and focused than she had been in months, if not years.

APPLICATION TO THE C-SUITE

Executives in the C-suite experience many of the same challenges discussed in this chapter, but the level of intensity is often much higher at this level. The distinction between high engagement and workaholism, particularly, can be difficult to see, and personal renewal often gets shortchanged. The following are particularly insidious in the C-suite.

The "Crackberry"

Left unchecked, executives' use of mobile e-mail devices can threaten their opportunities for reflective time. A *culture of connectivity*—an environment in which senior executives expect to reach and be reached by one another at all times—erases the natural breaks from activity during the workday. E-mails are checked during lulls in meetings or even conversations. The commute home becomes devoted to reading and typing, and a spouse's restroom run becomes a quick chance to clear out another item from the inbox. Senior leaders who display these habits are taken as models by the next level of managers; soon, they too are dangerously attached to their devices and diminishing their reflective time.

If you and your peers have fallen into this pattern, setting some limits can help. Some organizations have instituted informal or even formal policies against checking mobile devices during meetings, and they will liberally apply in-the-moment peer pressure when they catch their peers backsliding.

Off-Hours Demands

A senior executive is often required to attend off-hours meetings and off-site philanthropic/social events as part of her role as the face of the organization to the community it serves. These kinds of events have a habit of creeping up over time; last year's attendance at a particular event becomes an annual expectation, and new requests show up regularly. With only so many waking hours, these engagements leave less time for a home life and developmental reflection. Here, too, setting guidelines on what is a reasonable number of nights per week or weekends per month dedicated to attending organizational and community functions can be beneficial.

Overcommitment

Most senior leaders are overscheduled. For some, their full calendar is not enough; they also have a "shadow calendar" filled with secondary appointments in case the primary meetings get cancelled, get postponed, or end early. This pattern can give rise to an out-of-control feeling and is not conducive to a developmental atmosphere. To combat this tendency, some organizations have implemented strategies such as "Meeting-Free Fridays" and "No E-mails During (fill in the time period)" or made better use of meeting planning. Other institutions have experimented with sabbatical programs, and still others have placed serious emphasis on having their executives take time away from work.

Work Demands that Become Family Demands

Families, especially significant others, are expected to play supporting roles in the work of senior executives. They make social appearances at or on behalf of the organization, and they participate in auxiliary, volunteer, and fundraising activities. Such close involvement brings the job home in a major way, blurring the line between work and the rest of one's life. Effective leaders recognize the importance of their family's role in supporting their work, and the time and effort it requires from them. They pursue their family's involvement as a negotiation process, express appreciation for the support they receive, and avoid taking the support for granted.

REFERENCES

American Express. 2007. "Exercise and Business Acumen Linked; Genders Differ on Idea Generation." American Express OPEN Survey. [Online information; retrieved 8/1/08.] http://home3.americanexpress.com/corp/pc/2007/monitor_print.asp.

Church, A. H. 1997. "Managerial Self-Awareness in High-Performing Individuals in Organizations." *Journal of Applied Psychology* 82: 281–92.

Dye, C., and A. N. Garman. 2006. *Exceptional Leadership: 16 Critical Competencies for Healthcare Executives.* Chicago: Health Administration Press.

Gump, B. B., and K. A. Matthews. 2000. "Are Vacations Good for Your Health? The 9-Year Mortality Experience After the Multiple Risk Factor Intervention Trial." *Psychosomatic Medicine* 62: 608–12.

HR Magazine. 2006. "Exercise May Have Job-Related Benefits." *HR Magazine,* 16.

McDowell-Larsen, S. 2006. "Coaching for Physical Well-Being." In *The CCL Handbook of Coaching: A Guide for the Leader Coach,* edited by S. Ting and P. Scisco. San Francisco: Jossey-Bass.

Rode, J. C. 2004. "Job Satisfaction and Life Satisfaction Revisited: A Longitudinal Test of an Integrated Model." *Human Relations* 57 (9): 1205–30.

Westman, M., and D. Eden. 1997. "Effects of a Respite from Work on Burnout: Vacation Relief and Fade-Out." *Journal of Applied Psychology* 82: 516–27.

Wilson, T. D., and E. W. Dunn. 2004. "Self-Knowledge: Its Limits, Value, and Potential for Improvement." *Annual Review of Psychology* 55: 493–18.

The Developmental Interview Guide*

Section One: Position and Career Goals

Current Position

How long have you been in this role? _____

Ideally, how long would you like to remain in this role? _____

_____

What in your current role is working particularly well? _____

_____

_____

What are you finding the most challenging in your current role?

_____

_____

If your current role could be made "ideal," in what ways would it be different from how it is currently? _____

_____

_____

Future Position

If you do not intend to retire from your current role, what type of role would you like to move into next? _____

_____

_____

_____

*Note: You may access this entire form online at ache.org/books/C-suite

In what ways would you like your next position to be different from your current position? _____

_____

Longer-Term Focus

What would you like the rest of your career path to look like? (List positions and approximate length of time to reach each position): _____

_____

_____

Career and Organizational Setting

Please select the response that best describes your balance between career progression and staying with our organization:

☐ My primary focus is staying with this organization. I have no intention of leaving at any point. I will wait for promotion opportunities here.
☐ Somewhere between the statements above and below.
☐ I am evenly balanced between staying with the organization and career advancement. Although the opportunity to stay with the organization is important to me, if a good opportunity for advancement in another organization is presented to me, I will seriously consider it.
☐ Somewhere between the statements above and below.
☐ My primary focus is career advancement. I will contribute all I can while working for this organization, but my promotion decisions will be driven primarily by opportunity rather than employer.

If you think you may be interested in leaving our organization in the future, what kind of change do you hope to make in terms of organization (e.g., size, type, setting) and location (e.g., urban, rural, local, international)? _____

_____

_____

Section Two: Career History and Experiences with Leadership Development

Think back over your most recent two roles prior to your current position. Identify three growth opportunities (e.g., substantial projects, stretch assignments, development programs, mentors) that you think had the greatest impact on your overall effectiveness. What about these opportunities gave them the impact they had?

Growth Opportunity 1

Position I was in at the time: _____

What I learned from it: _____

_____

What made it particularly effective/successful: _____

_____

Growth Opportunity 2

Position I was in at the time: _____

What I learned from it:_____

_____

What made it particularly effective/successful: _____

_____

Growth Opportunity 3

Position I was in at the time: _____

What I learned from it:_____

_____

What made it particularly effective/successful: _____

_____

_____

Section Three: Current and Future Competency Development Needs*

The following competencies have been linked to higher levels of performance in roles like the one you are in and/or roles that would be logical career progressions for you. Before responding to the questions, read all of the competency descriptions in this section first. Afterward, you may answer the questions related to each competency.

Cornerstone One: Well-Cultivated Self-Awareness

Competencies: Living by personal conviction; possessing emotional intelligence

a. What feedback (if any) have you received on these competencies—as strengths and as growth needs?

_____

_____

_____

b. What aspects of these competencies do you find the most personally challenging?

_____

_____

_____

c. What experiences have you had that helped you the most in developing these competencies?

_____

_____

_____

*Note: The Exceptional Leadership competency model is used here for illustrative purposes. If your own organization has a leadership competency model, you may use that instead of (or in addition to) the Exceptional Leadership model. Doing so will ensure that the developmental interview process is well aligned with your other human resources processes.

Cornerstone Two: Compelling Vision

Competencies: Being visionary; communicating vision; earning loyalty and trust

a. What feedback (if any) have you received on these competencies—as strengths and as growth needs?

_____

_____

_____

b. What aspects of these competencies do you find the most personally challenging?

_____

_____

_____

c. What experiences have you had that helped you the most in developing these competencies?

_____

_____

_____

Cornerstone Three: A Real Way with People

Competencies: Listening like you mean it; giving feedback; mentoring others; developing teams; energizing staff

a. What feedback (if any) have you received on these competencies—as strengths and as growth needs?

_____

_____

_____

b. What aspects of these competencies do you find the most personally challenging?

_____

_____

_____

c. What experiences have you had that helped you the most in developing these competencies?

_____

_____

_____

Cornerstone Four: Masterful Execution

Competencies: Generating informal power; building consensus; making decisions; driving results; stimulating creativity; cultivating adaptability

a. What feedback (if any) have you received on these competencies—as strengths and as growth needs?

_____

_____

_____

b. What aspects of these competencies do you find the most personally challenging?

_____

_____

_____

c. What experiences have you had that helped you the most in developing these competencies?

_____

_____

_____

Summary

As a last step in Section Three, reread your notes. Identify three to five competencies that you believe you have developed the most proficiency in (with 1 being the most proficient). Identify three to five competencies that you believe you have had the least exposure to or need additional experience in. In coming up with your priority competencies, you should consider _both_ your experiences and the feedback you have received from others about this competency (e.g., through performance appraisals, employee surveys, 360-degree feedback, previous developmental assessments).

The competencies I believe I have developed the most proficiency in (list three to five): _____

_____

_____

_____

_____

_____

The competencies I believe I have had the least exposure to or need additional experience in (list three to five): _____

_____

_____

_____

_____

_____

Section Four: Development Plan
(Project/Assignment-Driven Approach)

Section Four should be filled out in collaboration with your superior, mentor, or coach after you have discussed your responses to the prior sections. Multiple copies of this page may be used if more than one project/assignment will be crafted.

Project/assignment title: _____

1. Description: _____

_____

2. Goals: _____

_____

3. Time frame (approximate): Start: _____ Finish: _____

4. Project contact(s)/sponsors: _____

_____

5. Skills/competencies for development: _____

_____

6a. From whom will development feedback be collected? _____

_____

6b. How will feedback be collected (e.g., employee/customer surveys, 360-degree feedback, formal or informal feedback sessions)? By whom? When? How often? _____

_____

_____

7. Developmental resources (e.g., mentors, consultants, courses, books): _____

_____

8. When will we check in on progress? How frequently? List specific dates or milestones: _____

_____

Section Four: Development Plan
(Competency-Driven Approach)

Section Four should be filled out in collaboration with your superior, mentor, or coach after you have discussed your responses to the prior sections. Multiple copies of this page may be used if more than one competency will receive focused development.

Competency/competencies of focus: _____

_____

1. Goals for the coming period: _____

_____

2. Time frame (approximate): Start: _____ Finish: _____

3. Projects/work activities that will build these competencies: ____

_____

4. From whom will development feedback be collected? _____

_____

5. How will feedback be collected (e.g., employee/customer surveys, 360-degree feedback, formal or informal feedback sessions)? By whom? When? How often? _____

_____

_____

_____

6. Developmental resources (e.g., mentors, consultants, courses, books): _____

_____

_____

7. When will we check in on progress? How frequently? List specific dates or milestones: _____

_____

_____

_____

Examples of Work Assignments that Build Competencies

The grid on the following pages describes assignments that can be helpful in developing specific competencies. These assignments work particularly well when the person is matched with an effective mentor or role model, and when the person is given feedback on specific development areas.

	I. Well-Cultivated Self-Awareness		II. Compelling Vision			III. A Real Way with People					IV. Masterful Execution					
	Living by personal conviction	Possessing emotional intelligence	Being visionary	Communicating vision	Earning loyalty/trust	Listening like you mean it	Giving feedback	Mentoring others	Developing teams	Energizing staff	Generating informal power	Building consensus	Making decisions	Driving results	Stimulating creativity	Cultivating adaptability
Supervision/mentoring assignments: assuming responsibility for student interns or fellows; having administrative supervision of staff and conducting a 360-degree feedback		☆				☆	☆	☆		☆						
Start-up assignments: starting and implementing a substantial new initiative, service, or product line			☆	☆	☆			☆		☆	☆	☆	☆	☆	☆	

	Repair assignments: addressing problems that someone else created in a division, department, or process	Task force assignments: leading a group toward achievement of a specific performance improvement over a finite period of time	Restructuring/reengineering assignments: substantially changing staffing or resource allocation to a particular area	Strategic planning assignments: assessing a particular area's current status and future options	Business case assignments: examining the feasibility of a new service or organization; proposing a plan for its implementation	Board service: serving on the board of a community or for-profit organization
1	☆			☆		
2		☆		☆		
3	☆	☆	☆			
4	☆	☆	☆		☆	☆
5	☆	☆			☆	☆
6		☆				
7	☆	☆				
8	☆	☆				
9	☆					☆
10	☆	☆		☆	☆	☆
11		☆				
12				☆	☆	☆
13			☆	☆		
14				☆	☆	
15			☆			
16	☆		☆			☆

Continuing Education Providers for Healthcare Leaders

Professional Association Providers

American College of Healthcare Executives (ACHE)
www.ache.org
ACHE has more than 30,000 members, including a large international member base, and a substantial regional chapter structure. In addition to its annual meeting, ACHE offers regional workshops, online seminars, webinars, and self-study courses as well as a credentialing process leading to board certification as an ACHE Fellow.

American College of Physician Executives (ACPE)
www.acpe.org
A well-established membership organization for physician leaders, ACPE lists more than 10,000 members, primarily in the United States. This organization presents regional institutes ("live programs") as well as distance education and on-site programs, many of which meet the academic requirements for board certification in medical management (CPE).

American Hospital Association, Personal Membership Groups (PMGs)
www.aha.org
The American Hospital Association has more than a dozen PMGs, each of which offers specialized development programming for healthcare leaders with specific interests or working in specific

functional areas (e.g., environmental services, human resource administration, risk management, strategy).

American Organization of Nurse Executives (AONE)
www.aone.org
A subsidiary of the American Hospital Association, AONE is the leading national organization of nurse leaders, with more than 6,000 members. AONE offers an annual national conference, workshops, e-learning, and accredited programs that target different levels of nurse leadership.

Healthcare Financial Management Association (HFMA)
www.hfma.org
With more than 35,000 members, HFMA is the United States' leading membership organization for healthcare financial management executives and leaders. This organization produces a national conference, regional conferences, and webinars. It also offers programs that can be delivered on site.

Healthcare Information and Management Systems Society (HIMSS)
www.himss.org
The focus of HIMSS is on "providing global leadership for the optimal use of healthcare information technology (IT) and management systems for the betterment of healthcare." HIMSS presents regional, national, and international conferences as well as audio-conferences and webinars.

Institute for Diversity in Health Management (IFD)
www.diversityconnection.org
Founded in 1994, IFD's mission is "to increase the number of people of color in health services administration to better reflect the increasingly diverse communities they serve, and to improve opportunities for professionals already in the health care field." IFD pursues this goal by offering diversity leadership internships

and educational programs, including annual meetings, workshops, teleconferences, "learning moments" case studies, and a certificate program.

Medical Group Management Association (MGMA)
www.mgma.com
The mission of the 21,000+ member MGMA is "to continually improve the performance of medical group practice professionals and the organizations they represent." In addition to its annual conference, MGMA provides seminars, online courses, and computer-based simulation programs as well as certification by the American College of Medical Practice Executives.

Private Organization Providers

The Advisory Board Company
www.advisoryboardcompany.com
Operating under an organizational membership model, The Advisory Board provides a wide variety of knowledge and educational resources to its 2,700+ institutional members, including on-site workshops and research.

Estes Park Institute
www.estespark.org
Estes Park Institute offers continuing education conferences designed to update executives' skills and knowledge of new and emerging healthcare delivery trends.

The Governance Institute
www.governanceinstitute.com
In addition to conferences and workshops, The Governance Institute presents briefings, white papers, and advisory services, all of which are focused on improving the governance practices of healthcare organizations. This organization also provides governance

support services, including facilitating board self-assessments and retreats.

The Healthcare Roundtable
www.healthcareroundtable.com
The Healthcare Roundtable establishes learning groups for experienced healthcare executives who are geographically dispersed at noncompeting, not-for-profit hospitals and health systems throughout the United States. Roundtables are organized around specific positions and functions, and these groups meet twice a year in facilitated sessions that feature speakers on member-selected topics.

The National Center for Healthcare Leadership (NCHL)
www.nchl.org/ns/programs/programs.asp
NCHL programs focus on senior executive leaders and leadership teams, offering mechanisms for participating organizations to share best practices in leadership. This group also provides consultative services for leadership development program implementation and support through the NCHL and GE Institute for Transformational Leadership.

Sg2
www.sg2.com/leadership.aspx
Sg2 is a future-focused research, education, and consulting firm that offers half-day and full-day courses through membership as well as custom on-site educational programs. In addition, Sg2 provides webinars, publications, case studies, and course "accountability" guides that can be used with mentors.

University Providers

Commission on Accreditation of Healthcare Management Education (CAHME)
www.cahme.org

Association to Advance Collegiate Schools of Business (AACSB)
www.aacsb.edu

Many universities offer continuing education programs. The quality of these programs can vary, but their costs are often highly competitive. Partnerships with universities can yield benefits, one of which is that they serve as recruiting pipelines. Both CAHME and AACSB provide listings of accredited programs on their websites, which are searchable by state and country/region.

About the Authors

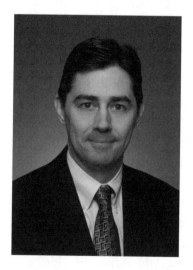

Andrew N. Garman, PsyD, MS, works as a faculty and practitioner at the Rush University Medical Center in Chicago. In his practice role with the medical center, Dr. Garman supports leadership assessment, development, and related high-performance work system initiatives. In his faculty role with the health systems management department, he oversees departmental administration and faculty development and provides lectures and courses on topics such as leadership, governance, innovation, and global trends.

Dr. Garman is a recognized authority in evidence-based leadership assessment and development. His research and applied work have been published in more than 25 peer-reviewed journal articles and books. For his studies of leadership competencies and CEO succession planning, he has received three Health Management Research Awards from the American College of Healthcare

Executives. He serves on the editorial boards of *Consulting Psychology Journal* and the *Journal of Health Administration Education*, and he is a reviewer for *Personnel Psychology* and *Leadership Quarterly*. A frequently requested keynote speaker and workshop leader, he also consults with executives and their organizations on their leadership development and people management strategies.

Dr. Garman's prior work experience includes a variety of practitioner and faculty roles in various organizations, including the Federal Reserve Bank of Chicago, the Illinois Institute of Technology, the University of Chicago, and the Illinois Department of Mental Health. He received his BS in psychology/mathematics from The Pennsylvania State University, his MS in personnel and human resource development from the Illinois Institute of Technology, and his PsyD in clinical psychology from the College of William & Mary/Virginia Consortium. He is also an Illinois-licensed clinical psychologist.

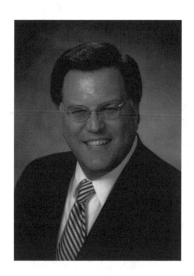

Carson F. Dye, MBA, FACHE, is an executive search consultant with Witt/Kieffer who conducts chief executive officer, senior executive, and physician executive searches for a variety of healthcare organizations. His consulting experience includes leadership assessment, organizational design, and physician leadership development. He also conducts board retreats and provides counsel in executive employment contracts and evaluation matters for a variety of client organizations. He is certified to work with the Hogan Assessment Systems tools for selection, development, and executive coaching.

Prior to entering executive search, Mr. Dye was a principal and director of Findley Davies, Inc.'s health care industry consulting division. Prior to his consulting career, he served for 20 years as chief human resources officer at various organizations, including St. Vincent Medical Center in Toledo, Ohio; The Ohio State University Medical Center in Columbus; Children's Hospital Medical Center in Cincinnati, Ohio; and Clermont Mercy Hospital in Batavia, Ohio.

Mr. Dye is a member of The Governance Institute's Governance One Hundred and also serves as a faculty member for The Governance Institute. He works as a special advisor to The Healthcare Roundtable and has been named as a physician leadership consultant expert on the LaRoche National Consultant Panel. From 1985 through 2008, he served on the adjunct faculty of the graduate program in management and health services policy at The Ohio State University. Currently, he teaches leadership for the Master of Science in Health Administration Program at the University of Alabama at Birmingham.

Since 1989, Mr. Dye has taught several cluster programs for the American College of Healthcare Executives and frequently speaks for state and local hospital associations. He authored the 2001 James A. Hamilton Book of the Year winner, *Leadership in Healthcare: Values at the Top* (Health Administration Press 2000). In addition, he has written *Winning the Talent War: Ensuring Effective Leadership in Healthcare* (Health Administration Press 2002), *Executive Excellence* (Health Administration Press 2000), and *Protocols for Health Care Executive Behavior* (Health Administration Press 1993). With Andy Garman, he co-wrote *Exceptional Leadership: 16 Critical Competencies for Healthcare Executives* (Health Administration Press 2006). He has written several articles about leadership and human resources that have appeared in various professional journals.

Mr. Dye has had a lifelong interest in leadership and its impact on organizations. He has studied how values drive leadership and affect change management. He is also a student of executive assessment and selection. He earned his BA from Marietta College and his MBA from Xavier University.